REACTI⦾N!

20
minutes
to live

REACTI⊙N!

20 minutes to live

Triumph Over an Invisible Enemy

MICHELLE FLANAGAN

**A world first journey back to perfect health and
FREEDOM from LIFE THREATENING ALLERGY**

REACTI⊙N HQ
PUBLICATIONS

Published by Reaction HQ Publications

REACTI◯N H⌒

www.reactionhq.com.au

Edited by June Saunders
Cover design by Michelle Flanagan
Internal design and typeset by Michelle Flanagan
Photographs of anaphylaxis courtesy of Michelle Flanagan
Michelle Flanagan would like to give a special acknowledgment to Karon Towns for her assistance in the writing of this book

A CiP catalogue record of this book is available from the National Library of Australia.

ISBN-13: 978 0 9872641 2 1
Australia

Printed in the USA
Charleston, SC

For My Family

and

In Loving Memory of

Eoghan

A Note to the Reader

A fellow passenger sitting in the waiting area of Heathrow Airport commented to me, "Once you get past the first chapter in the book the rest will flow."

His words about the writing process got me thinking. Do we all just stay in one chapter in life until we decide to go beyond the 'it' to explore? Then will the rest of life flow as we turn pages to other chapters? Writing is a metaphor for life as we go from chapter to chapter, getting past the first one.

Explore your story to recreate/invent your life. It will flow when you choose to turn to the next page.

We all have a story to wish for, a story that we create for ourselves. We have a cast of characters in our lives, there is a plot, drama—and sometimes conflict that can prevent us from moving forward.

We are the writers of our own destinies, the editors, and the publishers of our being. Our bodies are the outer shell or cover to a wealth of knowledge and experience within.

What is the content within you? Are you stuck on one page in your life, experiencing writer's block in your story, still on the first chapter but wanting to turn the page?

This is my story beyond the first chapter. It is my truth. It is my hope that my search is instructive to others in how to find and live out your own truths and write triumphant stories of your lives.

PREFACE

Imagine if going to a restaurant or having dinner at friend's or relative's was a life-threatening endeavor. Imagine that simple every day tasks such as brushing your teeth, having breakfast, feeding your pet, shaking hands with someone, or even greeting a loved one with a kiss might be the death of you at any moment of any day.

It was for me.

For almost thirty-five years, I fought an invisible enemy. I was a victim of Anaphylaxis. Anaphylaxis, better known as a peanut allergy, is the most acute form of allergic reaction; to date it has no medical cure and it can be fatal. Even microscopic traces of a food I was allergic to were enough to put me into shock, send me into a coma, and have me approaching death unless I received instantaneous treatment. At times, I had only twenty minutes from the onset of an allergic reaction to make it to a hospital in order to save my own life. At such moments, nothing else matters but to survive.

As a result, I had to live my life in a suffocating box, venturing out only after taking the most elaborate precautions and knowing even then the suffocating box could become my coffin. This daily dance with death meant that my approach to life was different than everyone else's. I had to do everything in my own unique way to overcome almost impossible challenges, each marked with the ultimate price tag. The true nature of Anaphylaxis is deeper than most other illnesses, as it is a condition that cuts right to the chase—sheer survival.

By the time I reached my thirties I felt like I had a loaded gun pointed at my head every second. Life was unpredictable, and the gun could go off at any time. There was no room for error, as the ultimate price was my life. Even those who loved and cared for me could become my inadvertent killers by missing the invisible enemy: in ingredients, on dinnerware, on the tablecloth, or in the food preparation area. One boyfriend almost killed me with a kiss!

Despite living with death constantly on my doorstep, I would see more countries than most people see in a lifetime; I would smuggle the least likely item across international borders; I would get caught with my pants down in a blizzard; I would be a first to legally challenge the airline industry to pave safer passage for peanut allergic passengers; I would survive the "Kiss of Death" on Valentine's Day, and I would find answers that defied medical science.

Ultimately, I am humbled that I'd become a world first to triumph over not only multiple allergies, but also "incurable" Anaphylaxis, early cancer, and an autoimmune disease. I did this because of a lifetime of suffering. It was literally do or die. Living a life scrutinizing absolutely everything just to stay alive was to stand me in good stead when it came time to understand my particular health condition and how to reverse it. At that time, though, it was a daunting task for me and mine.

Yet I found my way to freedom.

What was once believed impossible can be achieved.

I know this because I did it; I cheated death.

I continue to live without any type of allergic reaction whatsoever to date—and I even eat peanuts now! Some may say, "Big deal—she can eat peanuts!" But this achievement was so much more than that. Without death constantly on my doorstep, I could finally live. All was achieved using no drugs whatsoever and never coming into contact with potentially deadly allergens. The difference was that my focus had turned to resolving the problem rather than resigning myself to it.

But *Reaction! 20 Minutes to Live* is about so much more than just Anaphylaxis. It is about triumph in spite of unimaginable obstacles. Anyone who has ever felt boxed in by invisible challenges, anyone who has ever been anxious, depressed, lonely or addicted to substances, anyone who has suffered from post traumatic stress, immunological disorders, or other shadowy maladies will gain a new perspective on his or her plight. Anyone consciously walking their own healing path will gain insights and a roadmap. Doctors and therapists will also gain a better understanding from reading this book as it takes you on a triumphant journey from ill health to wellness, from despair to freedom, from turmoil within to peace without. It is an inspirational story for all who face what seem like insurmountable obstacles.

For some, the experiences I've written about may seem private, some may be difficult to believe, some shocking, and some may make you laugh. Often finding humor amidst the most unforgiving of situations helped me to cope beyond despair. Therefore, any humor in this book is not intended to offend, but rather to show how I coped from day-to-day, living with a serious health condition.

I have recalled my memories as best as I can, especially because memory is often lost or distorted during times of extreme stress or trauma. Others may remember events differently. The stories therein are my truth recollected from actual real-life events. Some have been documented in hospital records, medical files, test results, legal documents, and in interviews on television, radio, and in magazine articles. Also, I have more recent medical certificates which state I am *"no longer anaphylactic"*, that the autoimmune disease is in remission (a doctor's term to say it is undetectable), and the threat of cancer has never returned. Where relevant, extracts from five years of personal journals have been included. Any story from before I was born or when I was too young to recall have been well researched. I've also elected to change the names of, or omit, most of the people, businesses, and institutions depicted, to protect their privacy.

It is also important to mention that I do not proclaim a cure for Anaphylaxis. I am not a medical doctor or medical researcher; I am not even a scientist. I have extensive knowledge on this subject because I gathered it over a lifetime, seeking a way to live my life without having a life-threatening allergic reaction. I wrote this book to show the path I took on my journey to heal my life, but it is each individual's journey. I'm just providing some guideposts.

My particular case had become extreme; I know my increased sensitivities could have been avoided if more knowledge about the true nature of Anaphylaxis was known. That is one of my reasons for writing this book. After every anaphylactic episode, I was growing more and more sensitive to microscopic amounts of risky allergens, making avoidance almost impossible. It was literally life or death for me to find the answers. I share my path to conquering this condition in the hope that others do not have to suffer as I did.

If you come with me on this journey, a word of warning is in order: Anaphylaxis is a life-threatening condition with the potential to strike at any time, and it can be fatal. With Anaphylaxis, safety is of the utmost concern. The safety and wellbeing of yourself and others should always be kept as the number one priority. Always seek qualified medical advice, as the information in this book is not meant to take the place of a physician or any other medical advice. I do not promise or guarantee a cure, but I tell my truth about what has worked for me, to be used for educational or research purposes, or as a stepping stone on your own healing journey.

Under any circumstances whatsoever should you put yourself or others at risk with allergens that can cause an allergic reaction and potentially lead to an emergency situation or even death. It has taken me years of research, numerous bloods tests, and food challenges in a controlled hospital environment under the supervision of medical professionals to get to where I am today. Safety to self and others has always been of the utmost importance to ensure my survival, and I urge that you also follow the same path: keep yourself and others safe.

I hope that by sharing my truth you may benefit from what I have learned on my journey.

Michelle Flanagan

1

From the Beginning

"A beginning is only the start of a journey to another beginning."

Anonymous

I entered this life perfectly healthy, like a blank canvas ready to take on the experiences of life. Like most newborns, I arrived like a pure diamond that shone brightly at the world, without any apparent health issues whatsoever. The allergies would develop later. Yet the circumstances of my birth were unusual. I was literally born in a box.

"Good morning, Ireland," transmitted the radio next to my parents' bed. "The time is now eight-twenty on this cold February morning. A northerly breeze has brought snow showers to many parts of the country. Remember to take your time when you venture outside, and please stay safe."

"Put the kettle on," my mum cried from the small toilet next to the main bedroom. This request was typical on a cold winter's day, but a unique sense of urgency could be heard in her voice.

Without batting an eyelid, my dad climbed out of the bed into the crisp cold air, making his way to the adjoining bathroom to carry out his usual morning grooming ritual. Impeccable appearance was a must in the business world in 1969, and my dad was a master at it. Even if there was mayhem on the inside, appearance on the outside would tell a different story.

"I'll do it in a minute," he replied, looking into the mirror as he grabbed his razor and shaving foam from the vanity.

Outside the street lights still illuminated the suburban cul-de-sac, offering some solace from the long winter nights of darkness. The usual morning sounds were muted from the blanket of whiteness that covered the ground. By now most commuters had already left for their weekly avocations, and a temporary sense of calmness had returned to the street again.

"There isn't a minute!" yelled my mum, a pool of water flowing around her feet. "My waters have broken!" The inevitable was approaching fast, before its time and was totally unexpected.

"Don't panic," said my dad, remembering how long the delivery of their first born took, only sixteen months before. "I'll finish my shave and then make you a nice cup of tea. Just relax. There is plenty of time," he said, pondering his mental "to do" list for the day ahead.

"I need to go to the hospital NOW!" came the panic-stricken voice from behind the toilet door. "The baby is coming now!" she screamed.

"Are you serious?" he exclaimed, dropping everything. In seconds, he was standing behind the toilet door, his face covered in shaving foam, in total disbelief. "Are you sure?" he repeated trying to make some sense of what to do next.

"Y...E...SSSS, I'm sure! How can you even ask? You need to go next door right now and get Mrs. Hunt. I need help!" yelled my mum through sudden spurts of pain waxing and waning through her body.

In the 1960s, anything to do with childbirth was predominantly women's business. Men were excluded from the labor room. That meant that Dad knew only one action: Get my mum to the nearest hospital and quickly. This was about a thirty minute trip across town. There he could pace impatiently in the hospital waiting room with the other expectant dads. Mrs. Hunt, the neighbor next door, had agreed to take care of my infant sister and help my mum with the women's business on the way there.

Within minutes, my mum, my dad, my sister, and Mrs. Hunt were all packed into the family car.

My mother's request for Dad to put the kettle on now made perfect sense. It wasn't for tea, but to follow another Irish winter ritual: pouring warm water onto the windshield of the car on icy days to melt the ice before setting out into the cold wintry atmosphere. Once they got the ice melted, the car alerted the whole neighborhood of its departure as it screeched down the road toward the hospital.

They hit the early rush hour traffic because in the icy weather conditions, traffic moving in or out of the city had come to a complete standstill, holding it to ransom. The main vein through the city was blocked by impatient commuters, boxed in like sardines, stagnant and unable to move in any direction.

"Oh, my God, I see black," exclaimed Mrs. Hunt from her front row seat to my debut. "You have to find another way through this traffic. You must! It's the baby's head!"

My mum yelled, "I don't want to have my baby here! You have to move. Blow the horn! Just do something!"

Like an animal cornered in the face of danger and with only one way out, my dad improvised and launched the car onto the sidewalk. What followed could best be described as a scene right out of the movies. The drama was destined to intensify as they sped passed a motorbike cop, sipping his morning coffee outside the local police station. They passed within inches of his feet. It was inevitable that he would jump onto his bike in hot pursuit.

"Oh, Christ—not now, please!" my dad said when he noticed the cop in his rear view mirror. The panic escalated even more as the cop strolled to the car, seemingly in slow motion.

"Where's the fire?" he asked my dad as he glanced at the other passengers. Despite being hidden from view for obvious reasons, there I was popping my head out, as if trying to say hello.

"Oh! I see," he said. "I understand where you need to be. I will do what I can to guide you there, but not beyond my jurisdiction. You must take the final step on your own."

He radioed the hospital to give them a heads up on my arrival. And with his assistance, the path ahead was made clear. I often wonder today if he knew how timely and crucial his guidance was in my life.

"It is now eight-forty," the DJ announced on the car radio. "The next song is a very special dedication to all you commuters stuck out there."

"*Michelle, ma belle…*" Some relief was felt as this popular song by the Beatles began to play.

With the assistance of flashing police lights and sirens, they reached the hospital with only minutes to spare. Staff waited outside to greet and usher my dad off to administration and to whisk my mum away in the elevator.

"Phew! We just made it," My dad sighed with relief as he stood at the reception desk, wiping sweat off his forehead as he watched the elevator doors close. "Just in the nick of time," he thought, proud that he had accomplished his goal.

"Congratulations. You have a girl," said the administrator.

"But how can that be? My wife just left here about two minutes ago," replied my dad, bewildered.

"Your daughter was born in the elevator," she replied, putting the phone back in its cradle.

"On her way up, between floors," she said, smiling.

My mum had experienced what is known as a "spontaneous preterm birth", when the baby arrives before the full term of thirty-seven weeks, and labor comes without pain or perceived contractions. In most cases, there are no warning signs.

It wasn't long before my dad and mum were reunited, ecstatic about the new addition to their family. Despite the recent traumatic event, they were happy.

"What is the name of your new daughter?" asked the attending nurse, filling out the new arrival's paperwork.

"I think our daughter was trying to tell us her name on the way here," he said, recalling the song dedicated to commuters that played on the radio. Deep in thought, Dad's face turned a shade of pale; his eyes rolled upward and a sense of urgency filled the air.

"Oh! my," he said.

Mum braced herself. *Something was wrong.*

His voice spoke of disappointment as he explained the reason behind his sudden departure.

"Amidst all the panic to get you here I left your bag sitting in the driveway," he exclaimed. "But there's more...I also left the front door wide open," he said putting on his coat to take a journey back home.

I find it uncanny that the events surrounding my birth somehow mirror my life living with acute allergies. Daily life was surrounded by walls—boxed in by fear—trapped by potentially fatal consequences. Like a premature baby, allergic reactions came with little or no warning. There wasn't any room for error as the ultimate price was my life. The onset of symptoms was rapid. The window of time to get to the hospital for emergency treatment was minimal.

No two days were ever alike, as each came with its own unique set of obstacles. Planning ahead was always difficult, as every second was unpredictable and potentially deadly. Survival depended on constantly thinking outside the box, adapting and reinventing myself just to stay alive. It would take the next three decades to fine tune my survival skills, to learn to approach life in my own unique way. I would leave my baggage behind and find an open door that would lead me home, back to the bright flawless diamond within—to a time before my allergies and other health issues began.

2
Impossible Really Is Nothing
"It always seems impossible until it's done."
Nelson Mandela

At a very young age, I learned that no matter how difficult, unforgiving, or impossible challenges seem, the flip side to every problem is that there is always a solution. It's a good thing I understood this, for I was in for the ride of my life in a battle with an invisible enemy.

I entered this world at a time when milk and bread were delivered to the door step, mums generally stayed at home with the kids, dads spent long hours at the office, acute allergy was almost unheard of, and space travel sent man to the moon. On July 20, 1969, the world held its breath in anticipation as it watched the first man set foot on the surface of the moon. Cheers rang out in triumph and in awe of humankind's greatest-ever technological achievement. I was almost six months old when this wondrous event occurred.

Instantly, the word "impossible" changed to "possible". It became doubtful that anything once perceived as humanly impossible really was so. Even though I was too young to remember this day, it would have a profound influence on the rest of my life.

From then on, I was brought up to believe that anything was possible. In fact, my parents used to say, "There is always a solution to every problem. You just have to find it." This would ignite a burning drive inside me always to seek out answers, especially when faced with the almost impossible challenges that came with such deadly consequences later in my life.

My family lived in a modest two-and-a-half bedroom semi-detached home located in a newly constructed housing estate in the suburbs of Dublin. It was my parents' first house; they bought it as newly-weds. It included a front and back garden and was attached to the neighbor's via a single garage. Every house on the street was identical to the next, with the exception of different colored doors at the entrances. This was an important mark of individuality. Our door was fire engine red.

All the neighbors on the street knew each other by their first names, doors were left unlocked, and it was safe for children to play outside all day. Most days were spent playing games with the local kids in the cul-de-sac or in the garden shed at the back of our house. My mum's call: "Dinner is ready" was always the cue for my sister, brother, and me to end the day's play activities and return home, repeating this happy pattern day after day.

My early years weren't all fun and games, however. By the time I reached my fourth birthday, I had recovered from two operations: an ear operation to alleviate a build up of mucous in the middle ear, and the removal of my tonsils to relieve an inflamed throat. These seemed normal health complaints for a toddler—or were they indications that something else had gone amiss? I can still remember many nights crying myself to sleep after my mother flooded my ears with warm oil.

This marked the beginnings of a long history of frequent visits to doctors, medical tests, pain, prodding, nosebleeds, diarrhea, tears, trauma, rejection, and numerous admissions to hospital emergency rooms all over the world by the time I reached adulthood.

Instinctively, I knew that I was different from the other kids, but I didn't find out just how different and unique I was until years later. Also, despite always knowing that something wasn't right, no one had any answers for me.

With all the confusion, heartache, and frequent visits to the doctor with no answers, solace was found by seeking a positive angle on life and laughing at any adverse situation that came my way. To others I appeared to be sailing through life: a happy, chatty kid, who rarely took a breath for air from the moment I learned to talk. This outward exterior would carry through into my later years.

How could I have known as a child that my endless string of health complaints was not normal?

I had nothing to compare them with, but since my peers held no answers for me, I eventually started hiding how I really felt. I slipped in and out of my own little world, which I created for refuge, encased by a hardened outer protective shell that masked who I really was: a lost child disguising a ticking bomb just under the surface.

I was blessed to have an older sister to look up to and a younger brother to do tomboyish things with. Because I still had fun with them and continued to have "verbal diarrhea" (as my sister fondly called it, jokingly asking if I came with a battery or power source that she could conveniently unplug to shut me up) no one knew how much the health problems were beginning to take over my inner life.

Years would pass before science finally put a name to my symptoms. They were eventually confirmed as multiple allergies, some of which led to Anaphylactic shock, with the most severe allergic reaction to peanuts, shellfish, penicillin, and insect venom. Over time, I became so allergic to the above that they had the potential to kill me.

In my early childhood, an allergic reaction to peanuts and other common food was practically unheard of. Therefore, it's difficult to pinpoint when my allergies actually began, as symptoms often went unnoticed and were easily misinterpreted as something else.

This often led to a misdiagnosis, followed by incorrect treatment. For example, a runny or stuffy nose was often blamed on the common cold; abdominal upset on food that had expired; respiratory symptoms on asthma (the emerging childhood illness of the time); flushing of the skin on temperature change, etcetera.

The true cause may have been an adverse reaction to new types of food available in the market in combination with an accelerated shift in eating patterns. But beyond offering stereotyped treatment for the particular symptom, nobody was looking for a cause.

In hindsight, when I look back with the knowledge I have today, I believe that the first signs of my allergic disorder began to reveal themselves when I was about eighteen months old. It was only by the grace of God that I survived my early years without a fatal incident. I attribute this to mum's homemade cooking, with no canteen available at school, and then my dad's preference for plain, non-exotic cuisine. A simple home-cooked diet of meat and two vegetables was my family's meal of choice.

This simplicity probably saved me in my younger years.

By the time I reached adolescence, my symptoms were worsening. Still, I had no answers. I ventured out from the nest to experience life like any normal teenager, but I always knew deep down that I was different, driven by instinct to follow Dad's plain food preferences.

Of course, I took risks just to fit in—anything to belong to a group! I became a people pleaser in order to be accepted, and I formulated my personal identity around the outer protective shell that I had created.

I appeared to others as a joker, yet beneath the veneer my soul was crying. I was unable to make sense of what I was learning in school. The general guidebook for a normal life didn't seem to suit me. I did not know at the time, but every teenage risk I took was actually feeding the condition, making it stronger for future appearances.

Gradually, the reality that I could die if I came into contact with certain foods became apparent. Even minute traces, invisible to the naked eye, were more than enough to instigate an attack. Food that was harmless to most people posed a deadly threat to me, often sending my body into violent disarray, as if poison had just been infused through my veins. My innate survival mechanism did everything possible to expel what it perceived to be a threat, adjusting vital bodily functions to the maximum to ward off the perceived danger. I often felt lost and alone, living in what appeared to be an unforgiving world totally ignorant of the allergic disorder. This was evidenced by the lack of Anaphylaxis information available in books, articles in newspapers, or news reports on television. It was as if the disorder did not exist.

I remember being overjoyed when I found an article about peanut allergy published in a UK newspaper in the mid '90s entitled "50,000 people in peril". From that moment on, I knew I wasn't alone.

With the emergence of the internet and the worldwide spread of acute allergy, more and more websites started to display information about the problem, asking and answering such questions as: What is Anaphylaxis? How many people are affected around the world? How do I recognize a reaction? What do I do in an emergency? The internet became a great source of comfort and support. For the first time in my life, I belonged to a community that really understood my situation.

Yet despite the internet being a great source of information which raised necessary global awareness about Anaphylaxis, sharing and offering knowledge and crucial life-saving information, and bringing people together, I could never find anyone who had successfully conquered Anaphylaxis.

Therefore, any information or advice I found rarely went beyond dealing with the effects of the problem. This would keep me boxed inside the condition, living WITH it for many years until I started to look beneath a long line of effects in the hope that I'd find the cause.

I continually had to reinvent myself, adapting to an environment that wasn't designed to support my circumstances. I had to avoid allergens at all costs—allergens I could not see, which were found almost everywhere. To neglect doing so was to endanger my very survival. Yet even though this is still the allergy preventative method used today—avoiding allergens—prevention is difficult to maintain. Twenty years ago, lack of public awareness about Anaphylaxis made prevention even more difficult.

I had to check absolutely everything that I came into contact with. This meant that I was constantly reading labels, asking a partner what they had for lunch that day, watching what I touched or who I touched, scanning my body for signs, and monitoring my moods. My life was a vigil against anything that could cause a reaction as I fought this invisible, microscopic but fatal enemy.

Eventually, it became almost impossible to sustain safe living. Normal, everyday tasks such as shaking hands or brushing my teeth put me at risk.

People sometimes thought I was overly paranoid. They soon learned that my vigilance was the only key to staying alive. The possibility of an untimely death was all too real—and it was a possibility I faced every minute of every day.

As time progressed, my sensitivity to certain foods worsened, and so did the severity and frequency of medical incidents. By the time I reached adulthood, I was having an average of three full-blown anaphylactic reactions per year.

My body's response time was getting shorter, the symptoms were becoming more extreme, and the chances of surviving the next onslaught were diminishing. My body was learning from each incident, responding even quicker than before to what it perceived as a threat, increasing its power and volition with each response.

Gradually, I became a prisoner in my own home, consumed by hopelessness as my doctors told me that Anaphylaxis was incurable.

I would not grow out of it. It would not go away on its own.

There was no cure.

This was confirmed by another series of medical tests in 1998. Even though numerous doctors wished me well, they concluded that desensitization to peanuts was out of the question, and in my extreme case, there was simply no likelihood for improvement.

We believe so strongly in medical science in our modern day. Imagine what it is like to have a life-threatening illness that comes at you in the form of traces—mere traces—of common foods—and to be told there is no medical protection, no vaccine, no medicine, no surgery to cure it. All doctors can tell you is that you must be extremely careful at all times and that you must learn to avoid allergens to prevent death.

With few options open to me, I resigned myself to adapting absolutely everything in my life to suit my circumstances while I waited impatiently for the day when experts announced a cure. I waited and waited and waited, but this announcement never came.

Battling this invisible enemy was the only life I knew. The fight to stay alive was engrained in every aspect of every day. My allergies became my identity. How could they not? They infiltrated the essence of my being, even down to a cellular level. A person with severe, life-threatening allergies like mine can become defined by the affliction.

I had to become a master of survival, deciphering and fending off the enemy at all turns. I even had an anaphylactic reaction down pat, knowing exactly what to do when it did strike.

A life like this became normal to me.

I thrived on finding solutions for every challenge that came my way, especially the ones that seemed almost impossible to crack. My motto was that no matter how difficult, unforgiving, or impossible challenges seemed, the flip side to every problem was that there was always a solution. This belief became a big part of my coping mechanisms and my strategy to survive.

My focus lay solely on finding solutions to live the best way I could in order to cope with the condition. I never once gave the idea of permanently removing anaphylaxis from my life a second thought. Why would I? Expert opinion had imprinted the word "incurable" on my mind. I put my fate in the hands of science, hoping only to live around my affliction by constantly feeding its needs and demands.

That changed in 2004 when I reached a health crisis that brought me to a crossroads. Again, my doctors didn't have any answers.

I was left with no choice but to find another way, or give up the fight and let death win.

That was when I realized that my healing journey had begun long before I was even aware of it. I had traveled across three continents of the globe, and I had unknowingly gathered the intelligence required to win the battle.

On May 29, 2006, Anaphylaxis surrendered. I had finally won. This is how I know that nothing is impossible and no problem is insoluble. The impossible can be done. I know, because I did it.

3

The Modern Day Hunter-Gatherer

"Life is not what it's supposed to be. It's what
it is. The way you cope with it is what
makes the difference."

Virginia Satir

I became a modern day nomad, constantly hunting for
"safe" food to eat, instinctively wandering from place to
place in search of a better life. Every action, thought,
and motive I had were all based on the most basic of
human instincts: survival.

I lived from day-to-day. I lived only for each day, with little concept of
the future. Staying alive was more important than everything else. I
lived in constant fear, preoccupied by doing whatever it took to avoid
an extremely traumatic and potentially fatal incident. I seldom went
beyond satisfying each day's needs, and therefore rarely planned for the
next. In fact, a day never passed without my survival instincts playing a
key role. Life just seemed to happen, as if I were on a boat with no
oars, aimlessly traveling. I'd get somewhere eventually, but I would
never reach a destination of choice, except to stay alive. Somewhere
along the way, I bought into the illusion that I was in control of
Anaphylaxis, but in truth it was controlling me. Even though it allowed
me to expand my horizons as I searched for safe ways to exist, the
affliction always kept me grounded in the pure reality of my fleshly
survival. There was no time, no energy, and no room for anything else.

Every decision I made had only one goal—to stay alive. I often
wondered if my life mirrored that of our ancestors—the first humans
to emerge over 100,000 years ago—the hunter-gatherers. Like me, they
did little more than just meet basic physical needs such as find safe
food, water, and shelter. They wandered from place to place to find
enough food, and they did not have permanent dwellings. They
struggled to survive where other animals resided, and they were at the
mercy of an environment over which they had little control.

Was I a modern day hunter-gatherer and just didn't know it? Stemming from the first footprints set foot on this earth, survival is so engrained in our deepest psyche that if threatened, it will supersede everything in its path, making us wanderers in search of mere subsistence. I learned something about these hunter-gatherers.

Their habitat was plentiful in both plant and animal foods; dairy products didn't exist, and they rarely consumed cereal grains until the agricultural revolution approximately 14,000 years ago. They traveled most of the earth in search of food, prepared to submit to unfavorable conditions and to adapt their eating habits to whatever was available in the environment. They used instinctive intelligence to survive—a heightened sensory acuity with an innate ability to sense people, places, and things when the usual five senses of sight, hearing, smell, touch, or taste weren't enough.

I knew this ability all too well. With absolute certainty, I could instinctively tell if danger lurked around the corner. When the threat was confirmed, I couldn't explain exactly how I knew beyond all reason that it was there. I'd best describe this as a power of perception beyond the five senses. It was an unexplained power that protected me, one that was invisible, but which I instinctively knew existed.

Despite doing whatever my parents could to protect me from harm, they often felt helpless, and understandably so. My survival was dependent on circumstances in the environment, which could not always be controlled, even by following strict strategies such as reading food labels in so much detail; it often required a group effort. One change in a long line of cause and effect meant that my survival strategies constantly had to be reinvented to adjust to the ever-changing environment of life. Over time, I came to believe that this prolonged state of being in survival mode was who I was, shaping my whole identity. The mental, physical, and emotional impacts of living on the edge of life and death became my "normal".

So much so, I traveled to the U.S. in 1990 with a few college friends to spend the summer in Chicago on a student exchange program. I was twenty one years old, and full of bewilderment and curiosity about the world. Despite fear of a life threatening incident, I was grateful that my parents had encouraged me to explore the world before I entered my final year at college. I would later realize that Chicago was where I'd learn about the power of inspiration.

I can still recall walking down Michigan Avenue, savoring the originality of the buildings' architecture in the city famous for building the first skyscraper. I was in awe that each structure connected itself to the next somehow, as distorted images reflected in walls of glass surrounding it. Every day these architectural wonders had a different outward appearance, as every pane took on what was happening around it. They were continuously shifting and altering in guise, depending on whether there were moving clouds or clear blue skies, raindrops or the glare of the sun, shadows of darkness in the night or illuminations of street lights. This would inspire ideas for my final college project where I'd often spend hours downtown in the Chicago Loop, encapsulating distorted moments in time with my camera. But this wasn't the only place that I would find inspiration.

"Why do we have to do this so early in the morning?" I asked a new American friend, Judy, as I wiped the sleep out of my eyes. I recall that I was amongst a sea of women chattering while waiting in anticipation for the studio doors to open.

"I wonder what will be discussed today?" one would say. "I don't care…just being here is so awesome," another said. We were about to watch the Oprah Show live, lucky that by chance Judy had acquired a couple of tickets at the last minute to be in the audience.

Soon we were settled in our seats, feeling anticipation in the air before the show began. I didn't know but I was about to be touched in a way that would stick in my mind for many years to come, so much so I'd revisit it for inspiration when in one of my darkest hours. Lights— camera—action, as we applauded as loud as possible to give Oprah a big welcome onto the set.

The room lifted with roars of delight only to digress to a serious somberness when the topic was revealed: "Campus Date Rape." Over the next hour I sat in silence as I listened to the guests, young girls who spoke about their traumatic ordeal. Their stories of the ultimate threat and violation touched the most intimate of being, the private self. They were survivors of abandoned trust, hurt and anguish, when trauma had been dialed to the max and lingered to fuel more pain. I was inspired as I listened to the young girls reliving their darkest most private moments on national television, in awe of their great courage and bravery to expose the source of pain.

Even though at the time I couldn't directly relate to their experiences, an uncanny parallel resonated deep within my soul. I truly understood what it was like to encounter an extremely traumatic incident: to have your soul ripped apart in an instant, to be under assault by an unsuspected enemy, only to find out later that the fight or flight response leaves aftershocks that are just as, if not more destructive, than the incident itself.

It is to be left in a state of repetitive intrusion, thus killing any sense of what was once normal and leaving you profoundly changed. I wouldn't realize the significance of my presence at that particular show until over a decade later.

Returning to Ireland that fall, I graduated from college the following year only to find that Ireland's unemployment rate had reached an all time high. Gradually since the mid '80s there had been a mass exodus of young adults from the country, leaving in hopes of finding jobs elsewhere. The lure of possibility and a better future within one's grasp blinded many into leaving. My older sister had succumbed to the general trend the year before, as a fresh university graduate. Her destination was Germany. I missed her terribly, wanting more than anything to visit her after my final exams.

I was also a high achiever and made it to the top of my class in Design. Determined to make my mark in the world, I now refused to let my allergies get in the way of living my life. I can still recall the conversation I had with my mum only weeks before my final exams.

"I'm thinking of visiting Paula in Germany when I finish my final exams," I told my mum. "I've already proven that I can survive on my own without having a reaction, when I worked in America and Canada on the student exchange programs the last two summers."

After some thought, she replied. "I know, but you don't speak German. I understand you want to visit your sister, but I am worried. Not speaking the language puts you at risk. I really fear that you will accidentally eat something you are not supposed to and have an attack."

"Mum, I'll be okay. I'm old enough to take care of myself. Anyway, Paula will be there, and she speaks German. She can read the food labels for me until I learn how to do it on my own."

"What can I do? You are an adult. You never listen to what I have to say anyway. You will go, regardless of what I think. I just worry about you."

"Mum, I am the only one I know with these bloody allergies. I've made it this far. I have to get on with my life, and I can't let them get in the way."

"I've always encouraged the three of you to live your lives, to see the world. But your allergies really worry me. I want you to have the same chances in life as your sister and brother. But you are special. You can't just fly off to another country like they can. You have to plan ahead and be extra careful."

"How can I do anything in my life if everyone tells me I can't because of my allergies? You know I will be careful. I always am. Trust me."

"I'm not saying you can't go, and I do trust you. You are always careful, but other people make mistakes. And you can't afford to make any mistakes, because it's your life. You are going to a foreign country, and they won't understand you."

"Mum, there isn't a day that passes that I don't think about my allergies. I know it's the same for you. But I have to live with them every second of the day. You don't. People don't understand me here. How can they? They have absolutely no idea how hard it is to be in my shoes. It's my life and I want to live it as much as I can."

"I don't want you to go, but I can't stop you either. My hands are tied. Please promise that you will avoid taking any risks and that you will go straight to the hospital if you even suspect that you are having a reaction."

"I promise. I've managed my allergies since forever. Just because I'll be in a different place doesn't mean that I will suddenly change what I've been doing all my life. I'm only going for two weeks. I'll be back before you even know I'm gone."

Two days after completing my final exams, I set off on a plane headed for Germany. I remember looking out of the window with a smile, momentarily saying good-bye to the doom and gloom, chronic unemployment, and depression my country was going through at that time. With few prospects at home, I decided to extend my holiday to stay the summer, soon landing my first job as a designer for a large

European fashion house. Without even knowing it, I missed the family and country I had left behind. I loved them dearly.

Little did I know that I was about to encounter a significant event that would seal my fate. This tough life lesson would become the spark to ignite my healing journey.

4

Trauma in the Shadows
"Opportunities to find deeper powers within ourselves come when life seems most challenging."
Joseph Campbell

I had been in Munich for almost three months, determined not to let anything get in the way of my newfound independence, even if it meant not asking for help when I so desperately needed it.

I had become an expert in German cuisine, using food as my main topic of conversation. In the early days new people I met must have thought that my command of German was excellent. But I hadn't a clue; my vocabulary only extended to food. That was it. If "sauerkraut" or "wiener" weren't mentioned in the conversation, there had to be something wrong. I laugh now at the endless hours of boredom I must have put everyone through at the beginning, but to me the promise I had made to my mum was to learn to decipher labels. With my dictionary in hand, supermarket shopping could often take me up to three to four hours to safely read everything, leaving my sister at home while I disappeared to seek out words such as: *Erdnuss* (peanut), *Fisch* (fish), and *Schalentiere* (shellfish) that had been imprinted on my radar. But as the months passed, time spent at the supermarket lessened, so too did the yawns I received from others.

I can still remember the excitement I felt just days before my first Oktoberfest, Munich's annual beer festival, when a few million people of all nationalities pass through the city to imbibe the golden nectar, the finest German beer. I had waited in anticipation all summer for the two festive weeks to begin. I was full of enthusiasm, optimism and all the expectations a person might have in the early twenties.

The enormous tents filled with international tasters of the finest beer there is; the sounds of the Oomp-pah-pah bands wafted through air filled with the aroma of thousands of roasting chickens; the unforgettable sea of gray hats lined the streets; and of course, there was the smell of beer. The city was bursting with international flavors from all races and creeds, and all was friendly and inviting as everyone joined together in merriment in tents the size of football fields clinking their glasses while saying, "*Prost!*"

Almost every evening after work I met Paula and her friends to revel in the festivities. I hadn't experienced anything like it before and would never forget it either.

It was the last Friday of the festival, a night that afterward would come to haunt me. It was extremely busy. People were like herds of thirsty cattle desperately trying to get a drink in tents which were overflowing at the seams. We had been lucky to get seats despite the mayhem. When I look back I wonder if this was luck or all part of a higher plan to teach me something that I had been failing to recognize up to that point.

"Are you sure you don't want another beer?" a friend asked when I had declined after my second, a rare departure from my usual beer-drinking mood. Two weeks of partying into the night and working during the day had definitely taken its toll. I was too exhausted to get into tonight's festivities in a big way, but I went along anyway, afraid of missing out. I believe this lack of desire to drink to excess as I usually did saved me later.

"If the group splits up when we leave here tonight, let's meet at the usual Irish pub," suggested a friend, foreseeing that pushing and shoving through an ocean of people might separate the group. He was right. I lost my sister's grip by a wave so strong it forcibly disconnected me from the group, and I was left to make it on my own. But that was okay. I had felt disconnected from other people most of my life, so making my own way was something I could surely handle.

The uplifted drunken mood filled the underground train known as the U-Bahn. Oomp-pah-pah rang through the carriages as young and old sounded like a broken record, stuck on the night's most popular song. Laughter filled the air in what had become a very social network deep in the ground.

I was in my element. I reveled being around people, often going out of my way to talk to anyone and everyone just to make friends, to be a part of a group, to belong. This was survival for me. Connection is what defined my existence—to be accepted always muted the pain of rejection, which I had become so used to. If there was no food around, my mission to be included was at its strongest. I didn't have to enter into the conversation about my food allergies; I could be accepted for who I was rather than give anyone a reason to reject or leave me out for my differences.

I had spent a lifetime missing out on birthday cakes, social occasions, group activities, and other rites of passage since childhood. Unknown to me, a disease to please had been festering in my existence since childhood, growing stronger and stronger each day, built by layer upon layer of daily rejection. I would soon find out that this learned people-pleaser trait, when at its pinnacle, instead of making connections, had a double side that could endanger my existence.

"Where can we go now for another drink?" asked a guy sitting next to me, pointing at his non-English-speaking friends. My eyes lit up. I wasn't on my own anymore. I had someone to talk to. As the train passed from one station to the next, we got lost in conversation about the usual stuff; in fact I was doing all the talking. Where I was from, how long I'd been in Munich, how I got disconnected from my sister and her group of friends—basically everything there was to know about me, except my allergies. I knew my way around the city, and they didn't. The people pleaser within was shining at the opportunity to be seen as a godsend in the eyes of strangers, to make other people happy despite not knowing them, to be useful, even wanted.

"I'm on my way to the Irish pub...it's a really great place...you'll love it," I said, following a knee jerk reaction to offer to take people I had never met before there. Disembarking, I said, "We go this way!" happy that I had my own little entourage in tow. We went up the escalators and off the beaten track in the direction of the pub. I had taken this path many times before to avoid risk of an allergic incident. It was away from the main drag, which was laden with food stores and restaurants, so this alternative route in my eyes was safe.

But, through all my chattering, I didn't notice the demons from hell lurking in the shadows of this unoccupied, dimly lit street, waiting for the opportune moment to pounce. The people-pleaser had placed a target on my back, branded as easy prey to those looking for their next unsuspecting victim.

Before I could catch my breath to know what was happening, I had been dragged into an even more secluded, dark alleyway even more off the beaten track. The rapid pounding of my heart took over, washing out murmurs of people talking and laughing from a distance, my only hope of survival. My heart would become my only savior. I wanted to shout and scream but couldn't. How could I? My throat labored, constricted by a suffocating grip, struggling to catch my breath, sickened by the heightened smell of stale beer. Trauma sucked the moisture from my lips as the most intimate part of my being was exposed helplessly to penetrating desecrations from hell. I tried to break loose but the grip was too strong. Panic set in. A strong wave of revulsion was now coursing through every cell. I wanted this to stop, hoping that one of them had eaten peanuts and I would have a reaction—anything to take me out of this nightmare. Time stood still for a moment so I could hear the desperate screams of my soul through waves of pain: "Fight this enemy. You can do it!" I had heard these familiar words so many times before in the face of danger. But I had never thought in a million years that these familiar screams would come to me under these circumstances. Adrenaline began to pulsate through my blood, hidden power strengthened my muscles like never before. My inner thighs were throbbing, almost unable to move—but my life depended on action now.

"Move, you have to move," my soul was screaming even louder.

With a mighty lunge I broke free from the grasp of hell, and took fast flight back down the alleyway into the street lights.

"Somebody please help me!" I yelled from the pit of my lungs, like waving a red flag at a bull to get attention, anything to prevent pursuit of the tormentors.

All battered and torn, disorientated and confused, the sign of the shamrock over the pub door couldn't have been a more welcome sight. I was shattered. My heart, dignity, the trust I held for others, my sense of belonging, and the intimate core of my soul, had been ripped apart and raped of all essence. The long cardigan, meant to keep the autumn chills off my back, was now the perfect cloak of concealment as I walked passed the bouncer.

"Don't tell my sister what has happened when she gets here," I said to the first familiar face I saw. The emotional wreckage was numbed with shots of double whiskey. I needed time to gather my thoughts, work out what to do next. I couldn't tell my parents right now. This would only bring more heartache and pain from the bottleneck I'd already caused them. I had only been here three months.

"They have already been through enough," I reasoned. "They are proud that I have a new job in my profession…That I am making it on my own…I can't let them down," said the people-pleaser, rationalizing to have made it this far to prove that I could be independent. "I've survived the most extreme before. This is just another traumatic incident, right?" the inner voice said, convincing me to handle this like before, like I always had after being left to deal with the onslaught of extreme trauma on my own. The rest of the night soon became one great big blur as infusions of alcohol became the shovel to bury the demons deep in the unknown of my consciousness.

The next morning, I woke to internal cries from a battered and bruised body in pain, smeared with repulsion, repelling food and water, sobbing and shaking uncontrollably. Bitter stale whiskey outweighed the taste of the devil's lips. I was still in shock, yet feeling the familiar numbing sensation surge through my body with the usual thought "I'm still here" going through my head. There was an eerie familiarity about this feeling. I normally felt like this in the aftermath of an anaphylactic reaction. I was confused by this. I had survived an ordeal and endured pain that I didn't want to remember and I definitely didn't want.

It was similar to a lifetime of trauma from one allergic incident after the other. It could not compare to this monstrous wave—a tsunami of a different type—yet its aftermath was just the same lingering shock and a sense of surprise at having survived.

"I've just spoken to Laura…she told me you were attacked last night," my sister Paula said, concerned for my well-being, upset I had kept it from her. "What happened?" she asked.

"Should we call the police?"

"I need to go to the hospital now," I replied, pretending not to hear her, wiping vomit off my lips. My request was answered.

"They are going to keep you in overnight," Paula translated as she watched me deflate even further by her words.

"But I don't want to," I replied as an all too familiar pain began to bubble within.

"You are going to miss out on the party tonight," my inner voice declared. Despite being through the worst nightmare there is, the wound from missing out, built up over a lifetime, cut even deeper.

Even though my body was desperately crying out for help, a deep rooted part of me was trying to avoid the hurt I'd feel that night from missing out on something. When I look back now, I can't believe that I even considered going to a party when the only place for my physical and emotional state at the time was in a hospital. It just goes to show how avoiding exclusion can have such a huge hold on you. I would later find out why.

The next morning I awoke surrounded by about eight interns and the attending doctor. As he explained my case to them, I just knew by the wave of sympathy painted across each and every face that he had told them what happened to me. What did I expect? How could I maintain any sense of dignity or privacy when this had all been taken from me? I didn't care if he was a doctor or not, he had disclosed my most private details to a group of strangers. Ironic to think that I did the same to strangers if there was any chance of acceptance! His disclosure without my permission infuriated me.

When they left, the lady in the bed next to me whispered across the room, "I'm so sorry to hear what happened to you."

From that moment onwards my lips were sealed, and every ounce of my being was used to dig an even deeper hole in which to bury unpleasant things. I only knew that I had to keep this a secret from now on. Why, I didn't know, nor was I prepared to find out. Who was I trying to fool except myself by believing that I could keep something so big under lock and key? Something would eventually have to give.

The inevitable eventually did. Like a burst dam, I exploded the following year when the Oktoberfest returned. Smells of roasting chicken, beer on everyone's lips, sounds of Oomp-pah-pah, gray hats amidst an ocean of nations—this deadly combination contained just the right ingredients to release an almighty wrath of destruction from the depths. My deepest secret held under duress for almost a year erupted.

My sister was the first to be told, and then she told my parents.

"We have made an appointment with the Rape Crisis Center in Dublin," said Mum through the expected streams of tears.

"Your Dad is wiring you the money to fly home."

My torment was finally out in the open, relieved in a sense that the cloak had been put to rest. Hopping on a plane, seeing both of my parents upset, having an appointment at the Rape Crisis Center, would all prove too hasty and intense for my body to handle.

"I was raped," I said to the psychologist, finally snapping back to the incident in full sensory overload, down to the sick tastes and the smells. This sudden disclosure after a year of bottling it up proved all too much. The floodgates burst, and all hell broke loose. A dark cloud blocked the light and a tormented tsunami unleashed its might.

When I arrived back to Munich a week later, I can still recall the look of shock painted across my friend Catherine's face when she met me off the plane. We had met through the English-speaking community in Munich the year before. I connected with her on many levels. As if we were Celtic cousins from the past, her origins were in Scotland. She worked as a registered nurse and we socialized in similar circles. At the airport she waited with a wheelchair and ambulance ready to take me directly to the hospital where she worked. My body couldn't handle the pressure of being unable to hold any food and water down. I was reaching severe dehydration. The physical symptoms from the year before were the same, just more intense.

The hospital would become my home for the next two weeks. And to my surprise, I would encounter another traumatic incident in the form of NUT soup served there. How could the place where I was supposed to be cared for get my diet so wrong? This baffled me. Maybe by being focused on one trauma, they somehow forgot about the other. I will never know. Had I just done the same? Forgot? I knew that I had hit on something important. But what? This incident wouldn't show me what that was for another decade, when I was ready to look at this part of my life with fresh eyes, removed of the blinkers that had once overshadowed me.

Seven long months would pass as if I were a baby all over again— mixed feelings, tantrums, disconnection from the outside world, vomit and shit, confusion, inability to express what I was feeling in words and dramatically altered food preferences. I yearned to have one bite, to sink my teeth into something solid, but my body demanded a liquid-only diet. It had caught an eater's dire preference that only a baby on formula would know—tasteless fluid. If food wasn't put through the blender, puréed, or came straight from the supermarket aisle marked "for baby"—the only certainty was that solid food found the quickest passage out.

Was there a reason behind why my body had decided to reject solid food at this particular time? As if what I ate wasn't already restricted enough without this added hindrance? I would also discover no man's land, a place where memories had pieces missing—unjoined dots of information floating in space that when triggered or activated, created a living nightmare.

I can still remember the day when I had to go to a shrink for a psychiatric evaluation. It wasn't to determine if I was going mad, even though at times I thought that I was. It was to evaluate the best course of treatment for my particular circumstances. A lifetime of nightmares following one real-life traumatic incident after the next fuelled my torment—enough to drive anyone around the bend. Post traumatic stress disorder (PTSD) became a new label—I was an Anaphylactic with Post Traumatic Stress Disorder. This was the first time these two conditions had ever been married together, yet my doctors still treated each to their own unrelated to each other.

The psychiatrist's consulting room can best be described as something you would see in a movie; the comfy chair, a plant, a dimly lit room, wall-to-wall bookcases filled with mind knowledge, and, of course, the patient's couch. This was the place where I was supposed to divulge my deepest, darkest secrets—like those who sat here before me. And to a complete stranger I might add. Angered that I had to disclose the most intimate of my turmoil to a supposedly trustworthy and respectful stranger unnerved me, but the health system had insisted or they wouldn't help me.

"Blah, blah, blah, Michelle Flanagan, blah, blah..." said the psychiatrist in a foreign language into his Dictaphone, a small recording device. Why now? Could he not just jot a few things down on paper and write his notes later? This psychiatrist-Dictaphone relationship really ticked me off. When I was in the flow of deep disclosure in my own language, I was paused, forced to wait for his intermittent German mumblings to cease before I could speak again. I was growing angrier by the second. Every paused moment toyed with an internal switch that was about to blow a gasket. It only needed one last spark to ignite the explosive force within.

"Tell me about your father...how did he treat you growing up?" he asked.

"What do you mean?" I replied, not sure what this had to do with why I was there. As always, I wanted to please by giving the right answers, but this time I wasn't so sure.

"Did he abuse you?" he pressed. That was one of the many questions asked between conversations with his Dictaphone.

The fuse was short. I exploded. I couldn't help myself.

"This is nothing to do with my dad and you know that," I angrily replied, giving him an earful of my disdain. "How dare you bring my family into this," I ranted, disgusted with the psychiatrist for even implying a connection.

"I have just told you what happened…my parents love me and wouldn't do anything to hurt me…you are a man…is that it?…Just like those assholes who hurt me last year…or the doctor who betrayed my trust in the hospital…Screw the system…I don't care if they refuse to help me just because I failed this evaluation…Why should I trust you when I don't trust anyone else?…Trust…I don't even know what that word means anymore…I refuse to talk about my family…That's it…and stop using that bloody Dictaphone…I am here in front of you…use a pen or something…I'm tired of being put on pause after every sentence I speak…Do you not understand that I have been on pause for over a year?…Arrgh!" I snarled and hissed until time became my friend—time to conclude the session.

"How was it?" Paula asked as soon as I re-entered the waiting room. She was twenty-four years old then, and she was my tower of strength as well as my only physical support away from Mum and Dad. I depended solely on her to hold my hand regardless of whether she was prepared for this or not. This time I couldn't afford to let go of her grip—the only grasp I had on who I really was rather than who I had become.

"It was okay," I said, ushering her out so as to leave as quickly as possible. "He prescribed antidepressants and some other drugs that are supposed to calm my nerves…and I've to make an appointment with this woman."

I showed her a piece of paper hand-scrawled with the phone number of a local psychologist.

I had really felt like I had failed the evaluation but in hindsight I had actually passed with flying colors. For the first time in my life I had truly expressed what was on my mind—in this case it was sheer contempt. The people-pleaser was left at home and core emotions buried deep within had bubbled to the surface. Even though the prescribed drugs were a temporary fix, he referred me to a female psychotherapist, a Canadian woman practising in Germany—therapy that would span over the next three years. I would also receive a few months of speech therapy for a slight stutter that had materialized a few days after the incident.

With allergen avoidance always at the forefront and the aftermath of a traumatic allergic incident almost identical to the symptoms of PTSD, I wouldn't see the significance of the rape or everything else associated with it for over a decade later. How could I? I lived with trauma. Trauma played a sick intimate game with me every waking second, lurking in the shadows of daily life, waiting for the opportune moment to pounce. If I wasn't encountering a life-threatening allergic incident, every other moment was focused on the present, stuck in allergen avoidance so as to prevent an allergic reaction. Like a bad cold that refused to subside, I believe I had caught a form of daily traumatic stress. It couldn't possibly go away or subside when daily living came with constant reminders that death was always nearby. It was only a matter of time before layer upon layer would manifest into an explosive cocktail. I just didn't know it.

Five years would pass in Germany. Then, to my parent's dismay, I was caught on a current that would sweep me far, far away to the distant shores of Australia. I couldn't answer why, but the other side of the world had called. And the lure was too great to ignore.

Or was I just on the run?

5

Journey to the Unknown
"Often people find their destiny on the path they try to avoid"
French Proverb

Despite the limitations of living with deadly allergies, by 1995 I had crossed more international borders than most twenty-six year olds. I was about to cross another.

"Do you have everything packed for your trip?" my mum asked, breaking the uncomfortable silence. No wonder she was upset. I'd be far away from family support if anything was to happen. I made the decision to move to Australia—on the other side of the world— without thinking about the physical separation, the not being there, the uncertainty of departure, and being caught in a gap of time and space.

I called my dad at his office from the home phone. Most people didn't have the luxury of mobile phones back then, and if you were lucky to have one, it was often large, and it felt like a heavy brick in your pocket.

"We're just about to leave." I said. "We'll meet you and Mark at the airport in about half an hour." Mark is my brother, a tremendous support then and now.

I didn't know much about Australia, except that I had a chance at a fresh start in life. I had experienced far too much trauma by now, and I was desperate to get far away from the turmoil that had built up over the years.

The car ride to Dublin Airport was somber, making it feel like the longest thirty minutes of my life. I was afraid to blink in case I'd miss the familiar sights and sounds of the place I called home.

Passing a familiar shop on the corner, I laughed, thinking of the local shopkeeper telling her stories and rarely stopping for a breath of air; the pub culture with its many late nights of song and laughter spent with friends; the old buildings drenched in history, and the city center where I'd always bump into friendly faces.

I had learned a lot from previous travels and couldn't help but wonder what I'd learn on this trip. Every place I traveled to always had something to teach me—freedom in Boston, courage and inspiration watching Oprah from the audience in Chicago, fun and imagination in Disney World, safety and security in Toronto, design, languages, and food in Germany, the joy of having a siesta in Spain, exploring the past in the UK, and, of course, the most important, which was the unconditional love and support in Ireland.

Paula had since returned home from Germany. I was comforted when she reached out and held my hand the moment we turned onto the final road that led to the airport.

I felt part of a deep groove carved out of sorrowful goodbyes by those who had taken this lonely route of survival before me. It was etched in history since Ireland had suffered through a huge potato famine only a century before. Millions were starving, and survival meant to emigrate to Britain, North America, and the far shores of Australia. It was an ongoing trend, and by the mid '80s, emigration had become a big part of the Irish culture. In a crippled country, people learn to sacrifice, to say good-bye, and to do whatever is necessary to survive. Without even realizing I had become another in this pattern and chain of broken links to loved ones.

Dublin Airport was a hive of activity at Christmas time. With emigration in full swing, nearly one in every twenty people in the population had left the country since 1987. Among those who took degrees that year, a third of the medical graduates had departed, along with half the engineers and nearly three-quarters of the architects.

The arrivals terminal on the upper level was the place to be a few days before Christmas. It was a happy place, filled with many tearful reunions of sons and daughters returning home for the holiday period. Joy and laughter permeated the air, stories of overseas adventures were told, and never-ending hugs of love were expressed.

But I was in the departures terminal on the ground floor, three days before New Year 1996. The festive season was still in full swing around the country, but there wasn't an ounce of celebration to be seen here. My tears within wanted to burst into the atmosphere, but the situation was hard enough to handle, so composure was necessary until I had passed through the security gate to the international departures lounge.

"Can I have your passport please?" the girl at check-in asked while glancing at my extra hand baggage.

"I'm afraid you are only permitted to take one hand bag on-board. That's airline policy," she declared.

I could feel my eyes starting to fill with tears, but I had to be strong, especially now when the bag she was pointing to was the one that contained my food for the entire flight. Every time I flew, I brought my own food on-board, cooked at home to guarantee that there were no peanuts therein. I didn't want to take any risk, especially when I'd be 40,000 feet in the air, unable to get to the nearest hospital if a medical emergency arose.

"Ah! It's ok," she said. "I can see from your booking that you have a peanut allergy, have requested extra luggage allowance, and a special meal. Would you like a window or aisle seat?"

"I have requested to sit at the back of the plane, preferably close to flight staff. Is it possible to board the plane with the women, children, and special needs passengers? I would like to wipe down my seat."

"But the aircraft is cleaned before you board," she replied, skewing her face as if surprised to hear my request.

"I know," I said, "but I do not know if the person who sat there before ate peanuts. I have to be extra vigilant. I don't want to have an allergic reaction in-flight."

She picked up the phone and called her supervisor.

"That won't be a problem, Miss Flanagan," she said. "Please make yourself known to the ground staff at the boarding gate and they will accommodate you."

While handing the boarding pass to me she said, "Have a safe trip and enjoy your flight."

The dreaded moment had finally arrived, standing at the departure gate with tissues in hand.

It was very tough on my family, singling out each of them for a hug and some last minute words to cherish until my return. My dad was last, pacing up and down as if contemplating his words on his turn to say good-bye.

He is an astrologer and a believer in the idea that we all have a destiny in life. People would travel from all parts of the country to have their astrological charts read by him in hopes of finding their life's purpose or destiny.

"Michelle, I don't want you to go so far away" he said. "But I believe that we all have a pre-destined path mapped out in our lives. Obviously, yours is guiding you to Australia. And for whatever the reason, one day the light bulb will go on in your head, and you will realize why. It is part of your destiny to follow your path. Just remember to always stay safe, no matter where your journey takes you." He then told me it was time to go, the distress clearly seen in his moist eyes.

As I walked through the gates, I turned my head to imprint an image of my family standing there in my mind. I raised my hand and gave what would be my longest wave goodbye. It was awkward and upsetting. I felt incredibly guilty leaving them behind, as if I was the only one to break free from this torment and worry. I was the source of their hurt right now. But this was the price I was prepared to pay.

When the steel bird took off, I can still recall the heaviness in the air, the silence, as if weighed down with all my sadness, nostalgia, and uncertainty of return.

My next stop:
North America for eight weeks, and then on to Sydney for...
Return date: unknown

6

Up Close and Personal in a Blizzard
"Risk comes from not knowing
what you're doing."
Warren Buffett

I remember many storms in my life. But I will never forget the blizzard of 1996. Every city in the northeast, from Boston to Washington, went into a state of emergency.

The snow began to fall in Washington on January 6th. A series of snowy showers followed the rest of the week. Roads were impassable, schools and businesses were closed, snow ploughs worked around the clock, and many residents dug themselves out of their homes.

I finally made it to Washington to visit my friend Catherine who moved here from Munich a couple of years before. By now she knew me well, often by my side when the allergy struck. I always felt safe around her. She wasn't scared by my condition and knew what needed to be done when I encountered an emergency.

"I can't believe you actually made it here." Catherine said with delight, brushing the snow off my backpack.

"Yes, I know, the weather is crazy…and it's freezing. A warm cup of tea would really hit the spot right now. I am so looking forward to catching up with all the news," I replied.

We chatted for a while, updating each other on news of our friends, my trip in the U.S., plans for Australia, what it was like to work as a nurse in America, boyfriends, and anything else that had happened in our lives since we last saw each other two years ago. We had a lot of catching up to do.

Then the topic of my allergies came up. It always had a way of creeping into the conversation whether I wanted it to or not.

"I've been meaning to ask you something, but I'm not sure how to." Catherine said.

"My Irish friend, Marie, has invited us over to her place for dinner later. I told her about your allergies, but she insists they won't be a problem. She's really keen to meet you," She continued.

"You know how I feel about eating out. It's a risk," I replied, feeling a bit apprehensive about the prospects of not eating at home. I hadn't put much thought into anything beyond seeing my friend. I had presumed that because she knew my history, we'd be eating in.

"Yes I know," she said. "I suggest that we give Marie a call so that you can tell her directly what you can eat."

"Can't I just cook something here and bring it there?" I asked.

"I'm really sorry, but that's a problem. All the stores are closed because of the snow, and I don't have any food in the house."

Marie was a live-in nanny at the time. She looked after two young children and resided in the basement of her host's family home. Normally she wasn't allowed to have guests, but the parents made an exception this time. On the evening I was passing through, services were limited, restaurants were closed, and they needed someone to watch their two children for a few hours. Marie was excited she could finally entertain at home, as well as meet up with someone else from her home country.

"Okay. Can you make the call and let me talk to her?" I reluctantly agreed, feeling somewhat helpless. The allergy was so inconvenient, and it put me into so many awkward social situations like this one. At the same time, people just didn't understand because they'd never had a friendly dinner out appear to them like a death warrant.

"Don't worry! You'll feel better after you speak with her," she said, dialing the number.

"Hi, Michelle." Marie, Catherine's friend, had a thick Irish accent. "I've heard so much about you and can't wait to meet you later."

"Me too," I replied while trying to decipher where she was from by her Irish accent. "I really appreciate the dinner invitation, but..."

"Catherine told me about your allergy to peanuts and shellfish. Don't worry. We are having chicken, and I haven't used any nuts or shellfish at all. Is that okay?"

"It's not that simple," I said cautiously. "You need to read the food labels again for other ingredients. Often peanuts and shellfish come in disguise, written on food labels in codes, or under names you would never suspect. Do you have a pen handy, and I'll give you a list?"

"Ah! Okay. I didn't realize. Sorry!" replied Marie.

"Be prepared. This is going to take a while," I warned, grabbing a list from my bag. "For peanuts, you need to look out for: Arachic oil,

Arachis, Arachis hypogaea, and any type of nut such as walnuts, cashews, beer nuts…"

"I wouldn't have known." Her voice echoed from the other end of the line.

"Sorry, but there is more…The following may contain peanuts, so you have to look out for hydrolyzed vegetable protein, marzipan, hydrolyzed plant protein, food additive 322-lecithin…," I continued.

"Oh, my God. How can you keep track of everything?" she interrupted.

"It isn't easy, but I have to," I replied. Trying not to lose my train of thought, I continued: "Oh, yes! Salad dressing, nougat, cereal…"

I paused for a moment to take a breath.

"Thanks. I'll take a look at the labels again now that I know what to look for," Marie said, obviously thinking I had completed the list.

"Hey! I'm not finished yet" I said in a light-hearted tone.

"There's more…"

"How can there be more?" she asked.

"My hand is about to fall off."

"I haven't covered shellfish yet. Let me see…prawns, crab, lobster (langouste, scampi, tomalley, coral), crawfish (crayfish) …"

The list went on and on.

"The following may contain shellfish…seaweed, fries cooked in the same oil as fish, etcetera," I said, continuing to give her the list. "I believe that's it," I said.

"Can you not just give me a brand name and I can use that?" Marie asked, as if looking for a quick solution.

"Unfortunately, I can't, because food manufacturers can adjust their ingredients any time. Therefore, I have to check the labels every day whether I've eaten the food before or not, just in case the ingredients have changed," I replied.

"I can't believe it. I feel stupid I told you I didn't use any nuts or shellfish now…um! Now I'm not sure. I'll check everything again and look forward to seeing you both at seven p.m.," she said, closing the conversation.

Marie called another four or five times after the initial call, just to double check.

The neighborhood was affluent, populated by well-educated professionals, mainly commuters to Washington, D.C., who lived in luxury condos, or older style family homes. Thankfully, the walk to Marie's house was short. I didn't care too much for the sights in freezing cold conditions and heavy snowfall. Marie, two children, and the family dog waited with anticipation at the door for our arrival.

By seven p.m., I was so hungry I could eat a horse. The smell of food wafting through the warm air stole all my attention.

Given the numerous calls earlier, I was too embarrassed to raise the hidden ingredients topic again, so I delved into the food placed before me, ignoring all instinct to ask for a final check.

"Tell me, what happens when you eat something you are not supposed to?" Marie's curiosity about my allergy consumed almost all of the conversation.

I found myself drifting back to fond memories of dinner time with my family. We would all sit around the table eating the same food. My allergy rarely came up in conversation, and I could focus on the joy of eating, savoring the taste and flavor that was delighting my taste buds. There was no fear, only trust that the basic human need to eat would go as it was supposed to, without incident.

I was happy to answer questions about the condition as this raised necessary awareness about how to avoid the risks. Yet the more people I had to tell, the more my allergies became a constant topic of conversation in my everyday life. The constant conversation in my head was bad enough without having to repeat it over and over again. I couldn't afford not to tell people what I was allergic to; yet I couldn't bear the constant reminders of my struggle to stay alive either. Sometimes hiding away from the outside world was the only solace.

"I've seen Michelle react in Munich many times. I've even had to give her an adrenaline injection to save her life. Go on, Michelle. Show Marie your emergency pack," Catherine said.

I reached into my bag and pulled out an Anapen® (0.3mg Epinephrine (Adrenaline) Adult Auto-Injector), and small white plastic case, the type designed for a tooth brush. That contained a backup of adrenaline if I should ever need it. On the outside of the case, I painted a red cross often used as a medical symbol, inside included alcohol wipes, unused syringes, ampoules of adrenaline, anti-histamines, and a step by step instruction guide on how much and how to administer the adrenaline. (Today, the EpiPen® and EpiPen Jr® Auto-Injectors (0.3

and 0.15 mg epinephrine) are mainly used for the emergency treatment of severe allergic reactions/anaphylaxis).

On my right wrist I wore an S.O.S bracelet. When the top was unscrewed, inside contained a long piece of paper folded like a concertina. On it showed my blood group, list of allergies, next of kin, religion, address, and medications. Basically, it had everything there was to know about me. My bracelet was often the doctors' immediate area of focus when faced with an emergency, as it gave them crucial information about my medical history.

"I can never get lost." I said jokingly as I put the bracelet back on my wrist. "Do you mind if I have seconds?" I asked, still starved from not eating all day. "This is delicious. I've never quite tasted anything like it before," I added.

"Thank you. It's my signature dish and always a hit when I cook it," remarked Marie.

"The parents will be home soon," said Catherine. "We were thinking of taking you to an awesome pub down the road for a drink when they get back," she said, happy that it was still open despite the weather.

The two girls went downstairs to the basement to freshen up their make-up and left me alone in the kitchen. I didn't mind having some time to myself for a while. The constant conversation about my allergies had been a little bit too much to bear.

"Oh, shit!" I thought. It felt as if all of a sudden I had to go to the bathroom. And quick! It felt like a ton of bricks just hit my stomach. Brute force was an understatement to the almighty blow.

In the midst of diarrhea coming out one end, I had to grab a bin next to the toilet as a vessel for the undigested, mustard-colored vomit that was coming out the other.

The food was exiting faster than it had entered.

"This can't be happening," I thought.

For a moment there was a lull. It was the eye of the storm and a chance to make my way to the kitchen in search of the culprit. It wasn't my house but I didn't care.

I rummaged through the bin like a dog looking for scraps, looking for any clue to explain what had just happened.

"Ah! There it is." I pulled out an empty jar with mustard-colored remnants inside.

I knew that an allergic reaction was imminent. A storm was about to blow. With little time to waste, I hastily made my way to the basement. I held up the jar making sure that the front label was hidden from view.

"Marie, is this what you used to make dinner tonight?" I asked, instinctively knowing with near certainty that it was.

"Yes, I use that sauce all the time because it's always a big hit. Sorry, I cheated making dinner. I'm not really a great cook and wanted to make a good first impression."

"You definitely made an impression," I replied, while uncovering the front label on the jar for all to see.

"Oh! Shit!" exclaimed Catherine as soon as she saw 'SATAY SAUCE' in bold print.

"Where's the phone—I need to call 911 right now!"

"Is satay sauce a problem?" Marie asked. She didn't know that the main ingredient used in satay was peanuts. I hadn't included satay on her list, automatically assuming that everyone knew that satay sauce was actually peanut sauce.

"How wrong I was to make assumptions," I thought.

Catherine administered the adrenaline and called 911 immediately after. "Can I have an intensive care ambulance sent to the following address…immediately…My friend is having an anaphylactic reaction. I am a registered nurse and have administered 0.3mg of adrenaline…She has also taken 50mg antihistamine. All her vital signs are good, but she has eaten a lot of satay sauce…she has hives, swelling around her lips, diarrhea, and vomiting…"

"Ma'am, because of the blizzard an ambulance can't get to that address for about fifteen minutes," she was told. "There is a fire department down the road from your location. I'll send a fire engine to attend to your friend until the paramedics get there…They will have oxygen on hand if your friends needs it," explained the 911 operator.

Within minutes, sirens were heard outside. My rescuers had arrived—all twelve of them, decked out in full firemen attire. The dog went crazy as soon as he saw them. And so too did Marie.

"Do something…take her to the hospital now!" Marie yelled in panic. "Where are the paramedics? She can't die here!" she continued.

The dog was barking even louder

"It's all my fault…I should have listened to her!

"Oh, my God! Where are the paramedics?"

"Ma'am, you will have to be quiet. Michelle has to stay calm," said one of the firemen.

"Can someone please put the dog out?" asked another.

I remember at some stage looking through glass doors that led onto the back patio, surprised to see Marie's face peering back at me, standing in the freezing cold beside the dog. Even though it was a bit quieter in the kitchen, Marie's muffled screams of "Get her to the hospital!" could still be heard from outside.

The kitchen was well and truly crowded by the time the paramedics arrived. Just when I thought all the calamity was over, in walked the parents. I can still picture the look of shock on their faces when they returned home. To find total strangers up close and personal in their home, me a complete stranger with my trousers around my ankles, twelve firemen and three paramedics attending me, as well as one nurse, and their two children. Out on their back patio, their trusted nanny and family dog were going nuts, standing in a blizzard.

Suddenly the whole situation seemed hilarious! I knew I was not going to die this time. Catherine's quick thinking and the rapid response of the firemen and paramedics—even in the midst of a snow storm—had brought me what I needed to survive. I couldn't help but chuckle at the pandemonium all around me.

Thank heavens for a sense of humor.

7
Often First Impressions
Aren't What They Seem
"Life's a journey, not a destination"
Aerosmith

The world had become my university of life. My next course would take me further than I could ever possibly imagine. I was in for the ride of my life.

"Is this flight ever going to end?" I thought, looking at a world map and tracing the steps back to where I began. Only two months had elapsed, and I still hadn't reached my destination. As if caught in a time warp, it seemed like a lifetime had passed since I waved goodbye to my family at Dublin airport. No wonder. My itinerary read as if I was a celebrity on a world tour:

Dublin → Philadelphia → Washington → Chicago → L.A. → Sydney

Yet there were no crowds, no special treatment. No private reception would be waiting at the other end to greet me. Instead, I'd be arriving in an unknown world as an unknown myself, with no guidance, swept away from everything familiar on a self-imposed exile from my native land in search of—what, I was not sure. Yet, in a strange sense, I was looking forward to arriving at my next and final stop—Sydney, Australia.

How long will it be before I get there? I thought. I didn't know anything about where I was going, except through tales told by Aussie friends in Munich.

They spoke of their world: of restaurants, walking through Chinatown, having a barbie at the beach, camping in the bush (the Aussie countryside), and all things that make up the great Aussie outdoor lifestyle. Normal everyday experiences they took for granted posed themselves as challenges for my particular circumstances.

"Go to the famous Bondi Beach," remarked one of my friends, who reminisced about the sand, surf, and long summer days spent in the sun.

"Have a cold Aussie brew on me," said another.

"I'll definitely think of you both when I'm sitting on Bondi beach drinking a nice cold beer," I jokingly replied.

"We are about to experience some turbulence," the captain announced over the P.A. system on the Sydney-bound plane.

I was feeling more anxious as every moment passed. It was not from being trapped in this steel bird in the sky, nor was it from fear that someone might eat nuts beside me. Rather, my anxiety stemmed from not knowing how many more seconds, minutes, or hours had to pass before this journey would end.

Time was the only measure as to how far I was prepared to go in search of some stability in my life. I had purchased the cheapest ticket, taking thirty-six hours hopping from one airport to the next, on what seemed like the longest route possible to Sydney. Even though I was already far away from home, my itinerary gave the illusion that I was going even further away than in reality. I could have been traveling to the moon for all I knew.

Is all this heartache worth it? my internal voice asked, as I reflected over some sweet Australian wine, letting it breathe for a moment before I took the next sip.

Everything about my life was "over", I thought. Over-protective, over-controlling, over-concerned, overbearing, over the top...

Even now, now that I was starting my life over, I should have been happy, but I couldn't quite put my finger on how I was feeling. Anxious seemed about the best word to describe it.

The sound of a baby's cry echoed through the cabin, disrupting my train of thought. I watched the parents as they frantically offered comfort in an attempt to pacify their little one. But their efforts brought little or no success. Stress was building in the cabin; it was clearly painted across the parents' faces, amplified when other passengers woke because of the disruption, some showing their irritation visibly at the sudden outburst.

Within minutes, a flight attendant came running to their rescue, and it was as if she put the baby under a spell. The crying instantly stopped. The crisis was over. The stress and anxiety were instantly neutralized; calmness could be heard in the hum of the engines, and the muffles of others' quiet conversations were restored.

Everyone resumed what they were doing before, going back to their zone of comfort, whatever that might be. They retreated to their own personal space, to recharge, to recover, daydream, or take a break from the everyday stresses of life.

But I felt uneasy, constantly moving in my seat, trying to find a comfortable place to settle. I couldn't.

How could I expect to find a comfortable place here, when there was none in my allergic world?

How did I get here? Why did I leave everyone I knew, everything familiar, all that was comfortable?

I depended on other people for comfort, stability, to make sense of the confusion, to fill a void inside, to have all the answers, and to tell me what to do with my life.

"Be yourself and live your life," they said. But nobody told me how.

How could they? Most people didn't understand what it was like to live my life. Any advice shared by them was inaccurate or didn't apply to my circumstances. How could it? Their experiences were based on living in an allergy-free world. But I hung onto their every word, despite the inappropriateness of their advice.

At a very young age, I had learned to imitate other people's lives in my environment. Everything I learned in school or from peers was based on their general model of life. Instinctively, I knew that most of the lessons being taught were irrelevant because they didn't apply to my particular circumstances, even as I conformed to everyone's ideas. In fact, in other people's eyes, my world didn't even exist. This meant that there was nobody to teach me anything about how to live, or to guide me as I transitioned from one age to another.

I didn't know what to expect or how my life was supposed to unfold. Everything I was told seemed to contradict my version of life and its experiences. That's why I constantly questioned what was supposed to be true in society. I often felt stupid. It was as if I just didn't get it, but, in fact, the reality was no one could guide me but me.

The mirror I was looking at had foundational cracks in it. Vital information was missing—the information necessary to build a solid foundation. Or had I just been wired in a different way than absolutely every other person I knew?

I was lost, floating in space desperate to find solid ground in a world that had no solid ground for someone like me.

I became a follower, a chameleon, a people pleaser. I lived a nomadic existence, wandering through life on someone else's path, dependent on other people to show me the way.

I needed to fit in, to be included, to belong, but I always felt left out. I sacrificed my needs over the needs of others, and avoided any type of conflict, doing anything to please to make it okay for others, thinking that was the key to acceptance.

The yearning to be accepted, appreciated, and recognized took precedence over everything else—except survival. I lived in other people's lives, followed their rules, satisfied their needs, their comforts, felt their emotions, and solved their problems with little or no regard for my own, until that became impossible because of my allergies. My allergies forced me to find my own way.

Nothing was safe, secure, certain, predictable, or risk-free about my life. Therefore, I detached from my own personal space in the hope I'd find the stability inside myself I so desperately sought from others.

My life was spiraling out of control and rightly so. It wasn't mine. It was others', cut to a pattern that fit them, but not me.

I needed to find my own path, to get a footing in my world. But to do so, I had to break away from all things familiar. I had to go somewhere new. Start again. I did this when I left for Germany, but things didn't pan out the way I had hoped. My feet were itchy. It was time to move again—away from constant reminders of sheer pain and terror, the keys that opened a portal to the blackness within. I was too afraid to face what lingered in the shadows for fear I'd be swallowed in my own despair and couldn't ever return. But return to where? I was lost. How could I return when I didn't even know where I was? If people, including my therapist, got too close to releasing this inner blackness, I ran away as fast as I could, leaving the keys behind.

I can remember the excitement when I received a letter from Australian Immigration. Initially, I had applied for a one year working holiday visa, but after an extensive application process to determine my eligibility, a permanent visa had been granted. It was an omen. Hope had been reignited with the idea of a fresh start—a new beginning out of the silent depression I had somehow become accustomed to. For whatever reason, Australia beckoned. I could sense a greater power guiding my path—as if I were drawn to a light I was unable to see. I had to act.

"Ladies and gentlemen, please may I have your attention," sounded the in-flight intercom. "As we make our descent, we would like you to watch a short video about Australia's unique flora and fauna... and...please do not be alarmed when the crew move about the cabin spraying insecticide...it is harmless and just a precaution to protect our..."

Immediately my thoughts interrupted the announcement: "Did I just hear that right...insecticide...no...it had to be something else...am I just delirious from tiredness?" I questioned the unexpected.

Nobody had told me that I would be sprayed with insecticide in a confined space.

The video began and so too did the spread of an apparently harmless mist throughout the cabin as the crew walked up and down the aisles, spray cans held high in defiance. Any stray insect would surely perish from the dose of poisonous gas entering their lungs.

Harmless, the flight attendant had said. But, I had learned as a child not to spray cans in an enclosed space. Would it even matter if I asked the flight attendants not to spray? I didn't think so. This was outside my control, like the color of my eyes or being born in an elevator. I felt like a baby, vulnerable and defenseless in an environment shrouded in toxic mist manifested by the hand of another. I was tired from the long flight—my immune defenses were down. Forced to endure this unsavory air whether I liked it or not, I sat quietly, covering my nose and mouth, praying that the mist was as harmless as those who had implemented this protective measure claimed it to be.

"Out of the ten most deadly snakes in the world, Australia has them all," commented the voice on the video screen as images of snakes caught my attention. These were followed by images of spiders and sharks—more from Australia's most deadly unwanted list—as if the snakes hadn't been enough to scare me and any other new arrival. Until now, the only deadly insect on my unwanted list came with honey—bees.

Irish myth tells that Saint Patrick, our patron saint, drove all the snakes out of Ireland. Whether this myth held any truth or not, there are no deadly creepy crawlies on Irish soil. They were deadly only if you were allergic like me. Thankfully, pre-arrival spraying and the information video would cease a few years later. No wonder! Both were enough to scare the living daylights out of anyone about to take their first step in this country. It scared me.

The day I arrived in Sydney will always be imprinted in my mind as somewhat shocking, yet rather amusing. It was eight a.m., Sunday, March 3, 1996, when the plane touched down on the tarmac.

They say first impressions always last. Well, here goes with my first impression of Sydney and Australia.

I can still recall being caught off guard by the glare of the sun when I took my first step onto Australian soil, but that wasn't the only thing that had me captivated. Everything was bright and full of color, the opposite of the cold dark winter I had just left. It was the end of the summer, yet everything was still bursting at the seams with life.

"What a strange and unusual place," I thought, relieved the flight was over. I had made it.

The birds were chirping, but their song was nothing like what I'd heard before. They seemed to squawk. They were loud, brazen, and full of incessant foreign chatter—a far cry from the gentle, sweet, soft lullabies of the native birds in the northern hemisphere. Their bright colored feathers radiated from the trees, as if waiting to surprise the new arrivals with their strong Aussie accents and their unique songs.

The trees were also unfamiliar; some had flowers that resembled a bottle brush, while the wattle and the ferns, were consumed by colorful flowers and wonder. This was in great contrast to the bare branches at home laden with snow.

This world was definitely unique, an unknown jewel shining brightly, radiating on the other end of the earth.

I had to celebrate.

Bondi beach and a nice cold Aussie beer seemed like a perfect choice. I couldn't wait to call my friends in Munich to tell them that I had my first drink on them.

It was about a thirty-minute drive from the airport. As we went, I looked out the car window at this new experience, all my senses bubbling over with fascination. I found it hard to contain my excitement.

Yet as I got closer to the beach, the mad flurry of excitement turned first to bewilderment and then to shock. My eyes nearly popped out of their sockets when I saw the sidewalks laden with garbage. I was overcome by the stench of stale alcohol and the sound of loud music vibrating the car windows. The hair stood on the back of my neck. What kind of a country had I come to?

When I got out of the vehicle, I saw that the street lining the beach was chockfull of colorful characters. That was an understatement. In fact, there were men dressed as nurses, men dressed as brides, men in pink feathers and latex, men in speedos, in drag, wearing skirts and high heels and dressed in all the colors of the rainbow and then some. Women paraded as doctors, some were dressed up as grooms, some wore solid rubber ensembles…

Some people had passed out on the sidewalk; others kissed by the shore; others were dancing, drinking, and having a wild time. I watched this array of madness from the sidelines, stone cold sober, tired, and carrying a huge backpack.

"What have I just done?" said my internal voice, trying to process what I was seeing. The whole beach seemed to have gone crazy.

The Aussies are absolutely nuts, I thought, pushing my way through the crowd to a nearest bar.

"What can I get you to drink?" asked the barman, catching my attention with his casual dress. He looked like he had just come off the beach. He was wearing bright-colored board shorts, had sun bleached hair, and the remnants of sunscreen were still visible on his face.

"Straight double vodka," I replied, thinking of my Aussie friends.

I later found out that I had arrived the morning after the annual Gay & Lesbian Mardi Gras. The party was still in full swing when I arrived at Bondi Beach.

So much for first impressions!

8

David versus Goliath in the Airways

"Never doubt that a small group of thoughtful, committed people can change the world; indeed, it's the only thing that ever has."

Margaret Mead

The next time I would step on Irish soil would be at the end of 1998, almost three years after I waved goodbye to my family at Dublin airport. But to get there I had to battle Goliath, and it involved the coming together of a special group of people who would rally behind me to ensure that I got there safely.

The years just seemed to motor by, but ever since I had left my family at Dublin airport the yearning to be with them never had subsided. Adult responsibilities intervened, and three long years had sadly passed between hugs. That changed in October 1998 when it became apparent that a chain of family circumstances called for my presence at home.

At the time I was working as a freelance desktop publisher and illustrator for a chain of magazines published by David Koch, a well-known television presenter in Australia. Despite doing most of my work at my computer in my apartment, sometimes it was necessary to spend days at the office, especially when monthly deadlines were almost upon us. I loved being amidst a hive of activity, surrounded by journalists who had a finger on the pulse of world events. It was an environment I had grown very fond of. In spite of being a freelancer, I was treated as one of their own and was included in almost all of the office activities, such as the annual Christmas party.

The only exception was the occasional in-house celebration of someone's birthday. My reactions caused me to have to stand on the sidelines. I could sing Happy Birthday but I couldn't take part in the usual cake-eating ritual for fear of what might be in the ingredients or on the tableware. Now I believe that my working there wasn't by chance but was meant to be. David's team had come into my life to keep me from becoming isolated. But, more so, to stand by my side when Goliath appeared.

The emergence of the Internet gave me the flexibility to work online; therefore, I could take extended time off to go to Ireland. And one of my dearest friends Craig, a partner, ally, and tower of strength and support in my life at that time was to accompany me. He had never been to Europe in his adult years, so this would prove to be a real adventure for him.

Our tickets were booked, and as usual I notified the airline about my peanut allergy. I did not think much about this procedure of disclosure that I had followed so many times as part of the silent imprisonment of the box I lived in, protecting myself from death.

I can still remember my excitement the day we collected our tickets from the travel agent. These flimsy pieces of paper represented so much; they meant that soon I would taste home-cooked food, see friendly faces, hear familiar accents, and, most importantly, be with my family when they needed me the most. Little did I know that just days before departure all the excitement would be squashed into despair, which came in the form of unexpected news from our travel agent.

"Michelle, I don't know how to tell you this, but your tickets have been cancelled." Her voice was full of obvious distress at having to break this news.

"But…why?" I asked in disbelief, fighting to keep the pain of rejection from bubbling to the surface. Craig, in earshot, stopped in his tracks, knowing that something was wrong.

"Because of your condition…the airline has decided not to take you," she continued.

"But I told them about my peanut allergy weeks ago. Why now, just days before we are supposed to travel? This can't be happening. I need to go home," I said, feeling sick in my gut just thinking about the impact a stranger's decision could have. Someone was moving into our apartment in a few days; we had both put our jobs in Australia on pause, and I didn't want to let my family down.

"Can you call whoever you spoke with back and ask them to reconsider? Or better still, can you ask them to call me directly so that I can fill in the gaps about my allergy?

Maybe they don't understand," I said, still in shock at the cancellation. I was an established international traveler with no previous problems based on my condition. This was definitely a first, and what made the situation even worse is that Craig had been dragged into my world. His only crime was by association. He was being rejected for knowing me. This would only build on the anxiety I was already feeling.

"I'm sorry but their decision was final. Both of your tickets have already been cancelled, and there's no way of changing that," she replied.

"Can you book us on another flight?" I asked, feeling a glimmer of hope that I might still get to see my family in a few days.

"That's the problem. I tried to find you both another flight before I called you but I'm afraid there's nothing. I can't find another airline that can or will take you at this stage." She sounded defeated by all her efforts prior to this call. I couldn't believe it. Instantly, I felt even more isolated than I had already felt most of my life. This time I was stuck on the other side of the world. The gap between me and my family had suddenly expanded, and I genuinely didn't know when or if I'd ever see them on Irish soil again.

The reality finally sunk in. I wasn't going home. That was it. "This is really going to upset my parents," I thought, not to mention letting my colleagues down at the office. Literally, everything would have to be put on hold until I knew what was going on.

"Sorry, but I can't make it in to the office." I can still recall telling a colleague, apologizing for cancelling a meeting scheduled for the following day. Nothing but despair emanated from my voice as I tried to pull myself together to tell her what had happened.

It was as if she could feel my pain, her words of consolation came: "I'll ask around the office to see if we can help you...sit tight...it will be okay...I will call you back later this afternoon." She seemed as if she were trying to calm the torrential flow of tears washing my face. I had handled rejection well in the past, but this had cut away the core of my soul—my family.

When she did call me back, little did I know that within twenty-four hours a camera crew and a reporter would arrive at our apartment, the story would air on the national evening news, appealing for an airline to take us, one would come forward, new tickets would be issued, and the first of its kind legal case for peanut allergic passengers would begin. What was more, within days I'd be hugging my family at Dublin airport.

In 1998 only a handful of airlines had a formal policy in place to deal with peanut allergic passengers on their flights. This surprised me, considering that the main snack offered in-flight was a bag of peanuts. Something had to be done about the lack of policies in place, before something serious occurred in the airways—following the legal path was the only option. Four months passed before I returned to Sydney—a brief lull before the battle with Goliath really began.

But in my absence legal costs had been mounting and prior freelance work had since dried up.

Pursuing the legal route seemed impossible.

"Walk away and get on with your life," was the advice from my friend. "You can't afford the legal costs," said another.

"But if I do nothing what's to stop this from happening to me again or to anyone else? I have to do something but I don't know what it is."

I knew that my circumstance was an opportunity to do something about this issue, a chance to make a difference. I'd later recognize this as one of the first times in my life when I followed my own gut instinct rather than follow the path of others.

I began to knock on doors, pound the pavement, and make numerous calls until the Kingsford Legal Center came forward. I was thankful that they had agreed to take on the case at no charge.

About nineteen months later, the two airlines in question (I am unable to mention their names for legal purposes) agreed to reconsider their policies for peanut allergic passengers. Because of this case, approximately eighteen airlines finally took notice of the needs of peanut allergic passengers. In my eyes the case was a triumph.

The story would air on national television, except this time it was featured on *Today Tonight*, a program reported by Helen Wellings, who is recognized as Australia's foremost consumer affairs expert on Channel 7. Peanut allergy and the challenges of daily life would not only rise in Australia's consciousness but it would also reach the international stage. Over the next three years I would volunteer as the acting Travel Officer for the Australian Anaphylaxis support group. It was my chance to give back to the community what they had helped to give to me—the freedom to travel.

Even though my case was one of the first of its kind, unfortunately this issue is far from resolved today. Despite some airlines striving to accommodate peanut allergic passengers, others do not. This surprises me, especially when I learned from the American Academy of Allergy, Asthma and Immunology, that more than three million people in the United States alone recently reported being allergic to peanuts, tree nuts, or both. That equates to about one percent of the American population, excluding their travel companion(s).

I would also learn that under the U.S. Department of Transport's (DOT) rules, passengers with severe peanut allergies have been granted recently a qualifying disability covered by the Air Carrier Access Act. This prohibits discrimination by U.S. and foreign carriers against individuals with disabilities. But technically, DOT does not have the authority to change in-flight peanut policies. No airline can guarantee the complete absence of peanuts or other allergens on a flight, and the allergy policy of airlines lies in their hands. Yet in saying that, I have learned through my own experience that it only takes one to set the wheels in motion to make a difference.

What if beforehand you knew that on a particular day of the week you had to leave your nuts at home? What if one commercial airline took the initiative to offer a nut-free flying day per week or fortnight? After all most peanut allergic passengers I know carry their own food on-board, this suggestion would surely just let other passengers know. Would this not create a win/win for everyone directly or indirectly affected by this challenge? Those who wish for their in-flight peanut snack could still have them, while those simply wishing to make it from A to B without incident would get a chance to do so? Not only would a nut-free flying day minimize risk of something serious occurring in the airways, it would also give the growing millions of affected passengers what the community once gave to me—safer passage and freedom to travel.

Like any challenge, it only takes one to make a difference, supported by a small group of thoughtful people committed to change the world. I knew that I was meant to learn something from all of this, but at the time I didn't know what that was.

9
A Blessing in Diagnosis
"We can't solve problems by using the same kind of thinking we used to create them."
Albert Einstein

I had been told all my life that there was no cure for peanut allergy, aka Anaphylaxis. I was used to having an incurable situation. Then, in 2004, I faced diagnosis of another "incurable" disease, a Goliath of a different kind. Traditional medicine failed me, and I was forced to take my own path in search of answers. This new diagnosis would turn out to be a blessing in disguise.

"You will have to find another way," my doctor said as I sat perplexed at the thought that my body was diseased. I had Carcinoma. It was the dreaded "C" word. "The cell anomalies are in your cervix," she continued. The human reproductive organ necessary for survival as a species was literally under threat in me. I was in the preliminary stages of cancer. Why me? I asked myself. My body was clearly in battle against itself and I was on the losing side.

I had already been fighting my allergies, constantly checking everything around me in great detail. I had become an expert food label scrutinizer and a Grand Inquisitor of family, friends, and colleagues. I had to do that. I had to check everything, and I mean absolutely everything, just to remain in the land of the living.

Wasn't my existence already burdened enough without a diagnosis of early cancer added in? I already had an almost impossible task at hand—surviving when a micro-organism found nearly everywhere could be fatal to me. I was exhausted with the effort of trying to lead anything resembling a normal life, let alone one of authenticity, meaning, and untroubled relationships. Now, added to an already complex medical history, was the threat of incipient cancer.

"I can't believe it. Why me?" It felt almost surreal as I sat and watched the doctor shuffle through the multitude of pages in my medical file.

Deep down, I knew that the symptoms had been around for a while. If anything, this new diagnosis was just an official naming ceremony. As the doctor pursed her lips to speak, I thought, "Please don't tell me there is something else wrong with me too!"

"Michelle, there is a strong possibility that you might be allergic to the treatment," she said.

Now my allergies were standing in the way of my health again. I was in disbelief. They had already stopped me from doing so many normal, everyday things. But what was normal? Did I even know? Now they were stopping me from having treatment that could lead to my survival of another killer.

"What? I can't have treatment? What am I supposed to do now?"

"There might be an allergic reaction to the treatment," she said, as I listened to the details of an operation that would cut the problem area out.

Bloody hell! This had come at the worst possible time, when everything else in my life was out of control. It was hard enough dealing with the constant rejection my health situation seemed to invite. I was unique and seen as a high risk person in the eyes of others. One friend even said that I had an "ambulance complex", whatever she meant by that. Their lack of understanding often left me bereft of social activities, or else overly solicitous friends smothered me so much that I couldn't breathe.

By the time I reached my thirties, I had practically lived in a bubble, always in fear that I'd have a reaction. When I did venture out, nobody seemed to understand just how hard I had to struggle just to be there, because it was so far removed from anything they themselves experienced. The only ones who knew how hard my life really was were living on the other side of the world—my family. I wished more than anything in the world for them to be by my side right now. Yet I was strong. I had to be. What good were wishes to me now?

After all, my strength and perseverance to survive had got me to this point. Yet my world was crumbling inside me now. Any tiny glimmer of hope was still burning, but it was just hanging on, ready to go out. The years of constant battle just to live one more day had taken their toll.

I felt cheated that life could be so cruel.

"Operation! But I don't have any money to pay for this. I can't even afford private health insurance. Shit! Early cancer! All the symptoms I've had in the past have always pointed to allergy." There was still a glimmer of hope.

"Maybe the test results were wrong?

Had my obsession with my allergies masked that something else had gone into crisis in my body? Was there any pre-warning and I simply turned a blind eye to the signs because I couldn't cope with anything more? There had obviously been something else going on under the surface. Why had I not picked up on this more? I realized I should be grateful to the doctor for revealing it to me, as it was clear it was hard for her to break this news.

My life revolved around my allergies. They were my identity. Most of my life was spent focusing on them and only them. They dictated my behavior and they affected how others acted around me. After all, I had to be vigilant because my life was at stake. Life was a double-edged sword, even down to treatment options, or any other advice or help I'd receive from my doctors or anyone else. Mine was a journey through uncharted territory, with few people able to guide me. I followed the beat of a different drummer because I had to. The rhythm everyone else followed would be fatal to me.

"What I've never had, I'll never miss," my motto. The foods I couldn't eat, the friends I couldn't make, my beliefs, my future career and the places I wanted to go—I would do all I could with what was allowed by my allergies and never look back at the rest. My trials, I figured, made me stronger. I was used to dealing with trauma, not just from an allergic episode. Yet this news was too much to bear.

"Are you sure this is not a new allergy to something?" I asked. I wasn't going to let go of my grasp on the little hope remaining. I knew exactly how to deal with new allergies.

"No," she replied. "I'll refer you to a specialist who can tell you more about the operation. There is a four month wait if you go through the public system. However, it is free."

"I don't have four months," I thought to myself.

I was a survivor of the most intense traumatic medical emergencies imaginable—extremities that made me dance with death. Every day I dealt with the reality that it might be my last. I had learned to adapt to whatever life brought me by having a positive attitude. Even though my doctor's facial expression was daunting as she read my file, I knew that she was only trying to find a way to help me.

"Face it!" said the little voice inside my head. "Something is obviously not working, and you seriously need to address it. The doctor is trying to find a solution through conventional means. Your medical history is complex and a challenge for any doctor to find an answer. There is no precedent for your particular case. Wake up! How can she possibly find a solution?"

I realized I had reached a major crossroads in my life. Normally I ran away from a situation as far as possible. I had been doing this from a young age—avoiding facing things head-on. This was achieved by either looking down at the bottom of an empty beer glass or hiding, out of contact, sometimes for days or even weeks at a time. I stuck my head out only when I believed that the threat had passed and everything had subsided. I was the Queen of Avoidance.

This—cancer—I couldn't avoid. A rush of thoughts continued to flash through my head. My doctor became a blur through the tears that started to flow.

"Will you have someone there for you at home when you leave here?" she asked.

Yes, my boyfriend would be home. But I had learned throughout my condition that, in the end, it is you alone facing it. So, yes, someone would be home. But no, no one could ever really be there for me in facing my special health situation. I would have to be there for myself, dealing with it all alone, as I always had.

The diagnosis seemed dire. No cure had been found for Anaphylaxis yet; how could there possibly be a medical cure for an Anaphylactic with carcinoma?

I sat for a minute, trying to think of something funny to say, positive thoughts—anything to make light of the situation. I had followed this path since childhood. Yet my body was tense; I was fighting the tears, and my limbs were numb in shock.

My coping mechanisms started to kick in. On the outside, I was displaying strength, a total contradiction to what was really happening inside where I was falling apart.

My mind had switched to auto pilot in fantasy land. It told me that everything was fabulous. My body, however, was detached and reacting in a totally shocked and upset way. My mind was lying to me. It was doing everything it knew how to avoid the pain of realizing that I was not okay. The situation was anything but happy and amusing. My body was telling the truth, as always.

It was suddenly clear to me that my body was yelling at me big time. It was working on overdrive to protect me, and I hadn't bothered to listen to the signs. How and why did my body learn to fight against itself when I did everything possible in my daily life to stay at peace and prevent an allergic reaction?

That's it! I thought. My life was reaction prevention. My focus lay solely on this, which masked that some other part of my body was suffering. My mind and body were clearly out of sync. My immune system acted as the mediator. How could it possibly function when it was receiving mixed messages? It was doing its best to protect me amidst the conflict.

Now I faced another immune-type disorder as a result. I didn't know anything about this new diagnosis, nor did I have any time to find out about it. I was exhausted just managing my allergies.

"I will have to face the reality and find a solution beyond traditional medicine," I realized.

My allergies would become a blessing to me because they trained me to think outside the square to find almost impossible solutions in order to survive. I felt somewhat relieved. I knew I could do what I had done all my life. I had to search for the solution to an impossible situation. My body was challenging the Queen of Avoidance to face her situation head on and do more than damage control.

"Everything you avoid in life isn't all related to your allergies," my body was telling me.

"It is time to wake up and act!"

"I can survive my allergies every day, so getting through this should just be a walk in the park," I said to her, smiling, while trying to convince myself that this was just another bump in the road.

The sounds of oomp-pah-pah hit my mind like a familiar train about to wreck. The taste of stale beer engulfed my mouth, and my nostrils began to itch. I grabbed my nose to contain a sneeze. I began to feel sick to my stomach, consumed by thoughts that the most intimate part of my body was under attack again. The incident in Munich had something to do with this new diagnosis. I just didn't know what. How could I not have joined these dots before when the screams were coming from between my thighs? The tormentors of my past had finally caught up with me, this time bearing salt for my already festering wounds. The bitter sting came as a harsh reminder that this torment wasn't going away. Trying to ignore it in the past obviously hadn't worked. These ghosts were looking at me straight in the eye, demanding my attention: Face us or else you die. The message rang as clear as a bell.

I knew that to face the demons of my past required courage. It didn't matter how far I ran; if something was left unresolved it would eventually catch me. But it also told me a place to begin. "How did the girls who spoke on Oprah that day in Chicago deal with their demons?" I asked myself. Unknown to me, the girls had imparted their courage to me to face my own most private self of being.

The buildings in Chicago had inspired my final college project, but they would also teach me something. Could my body act in the same way, like every pane that shifts and changes as distorted reflections according to the conditions in their environments? Had my cells begun to distort because the conditions of the internal environment had changed? What if I changed these internal conditions? Would cell behavior change too?" I felt the glimmer of hope brighten. Had I just had a revelation? I knew deep down that there was a way to beat this new challenge. I just had to find it.

That's it! I thought. I've found solutions for almost impossible challenges. This seems almost insignificant to the difficult challenges I've already faced in my life. After all, I've survived death so many times. This is just another hurdle to overcome. My body, mind, and immune system were clearly out of sync, and they were trying to tell me something.

I took the referral letter from my doctor and departed.

Even though I still felt numb from this latest health development, I knew that I was a fighter.

This new diagnosis came like a baby's first words—the start of a journey to a new beginning. I now had a physical place to start. All I had to do was figure out what my body was trying to say.

10
The Psychology of Recovery
Am I Ready?
"No matter how difficult the journey,
we never walk alone."

Martin Luther King, Jr.

I felt alone and overwhelmed, knowing the enormous task involved when one puts her health under the microscope. I knew this from years of process-of-elimination diets and numerous medical tests to identify the allergens I reacted to. But what did I know about this new problem? And, given my circumstances, was I even ready for recovery?

"Create a list of all the professionals you think might be able to help you," was my doctor's request as I departed her practise.

But I had something more pressing on my mind. How could I possibly tell Andrew (my boyfriend at the time) that there was something else wrong with me? I felt awkward about telling him about an illness I knew very little about. I didn't want to be any more of a burden in our relationship than I believed I already was.

What if I don't tell him? I thought, knowing deep down the problem would eventually reveal itself. This was too huge to hide, and even if I tried to, the act of covering it up would only place a greater burden on me. Is Andrew going to reject me? I wondered, fumbling for my front door keys for fear they'd slip through my sweaty palms. By now we had lived together for over two years, and despite having many ups, lately our relationship seemed to be on its way down. Feeling like I was walking on egg shells had become more frequent; my sensitivity to criticism had heightened; and my self-esteem was at an all time low. But I had become dependent on him, and I was prepared to soldier on, no matter what, out of fear of being on my own.

"Do you love me?" I often asked him, as if to satisfy an insatiable craving for love and affection buried deep inside.

At some stage unknown to me, I had decided that I'd be "nothing" if I was ever abandoned, so I was constantly demanding declarations of love for reassurance.

As I opened the door and walked over the threshold, I thought of the day I first told my friends about this house.

"The realtor has approved our rental application," I recall telling my friends only the year before. "The house is huge—three bedrooms, two bathrooms, with a massive garden at the front and back." I remember feeling excited by the possibility of finally getting the space in my life I so desperately craved.

"But it's on the other side of the city," I continued, subtly breaking the news to my friends that I wouldn't be able to see them as much as I would like to anymore.

"Haven't you just resigned from your job? Isn't this all too quick and irrational?" asked one of my friends, obviously feeling uncertain about my decision to move away from the support network I had spent years creating.

"It's okay. I've talked this through with Andrew and I need to do this," I replied. I was a little confused, it must be said, because I thought making a commitment to him meant I had to make sacrifices.

"But how are you going to honor the lease and pay your rent?" another asked, as if feeling the vibration of uncertainty radiating from my being.

"Andrew is going to find me work designing websites through the business he has set up," I said, delighted by the prospect of working from home. Deep down, I had hoped that this move would alleviate the insecurity I often felt in the workplace. Despite the efforts of my bosses to prevent an allergic reaction, which I am grateful for, the issuing of a "peanut ban" without the proper training actually increased the risk, which had led to three severe reactions at work.

Despite my friends' apprehension, I moved anyway. The lure of space and security was too great to resist.

But gradually, over time, I felt isolated. I had no car to visit my friends, and eventually I became totally dependent on Andrew for everything. The bright chirpy person that I once believed I was had been left behind, and little more than an empty shell remained.

All my power and trust had been forfeited in return for work, food, shelter, love, and ultimately survival. The need to control the outcome of my allergies, coupled with the inability to plan beyond the day, made making decisions very difficult. Gradually, I became less assertive in making my own decisions, more inhibited and awkward in conversations for fear of exposing weakness and my low self-esteem.

Andrew had become my rock. By placing all my attention on the restrictions that kept my allergies at bay, there were little or no boundaries left for anything else. Handing over the responsibility for myself to someone else satisfied my not wanting to be accountable for the life I had not wished for. Now there was someone else to blame when things didn't work out, when mistakes were made. The idea of having a rock to hang my life on sounded like sweet music to my ears.

Now we were arguing about every little thing, arguing more frequently, and sometimes we wouldn't speak to each other for days in silent revolt. I found refuge in the bedroom, locking the door against the world to read books and write. Had I somehow played a part in instigating more and more arguments? Was I unconsciously creating the perfect opportunity to take the personal space I so desperately craved? I would later come to realize that even though I got my space, this method also brought more heartache and pain into my life.

"What did the doctor say?" Andrew asked as soon as I walked into the kitchen.

Automatically, I put the kettle on to make a cup of tea. In times of crisis, the Irish sit around the table together drinking tea for comfort. I proceeded to tell of my most recent health crisis as Andrew sat quietly and absorbed the terrible news.

Time stood still for what seemed like ages. I was smiling at him while I waited for his response. Now, I finally realized why I inappropriately smiled or laughed when I spoke to others about the traumatic events of my life. I genuinely had no idea how I was feeling, as if cut off from my body, with an uncertain sense of myself. It was a skewed coping mechanism.

"Oh! Michelle, how many times must I tell you not to leave tea rings on the counter?" he replied, grabbing a cloth from the sink to wipe the counter down in a furious fit. His display of frustration emanated a message of disapproval to the people pleaser within me.

This response was enough to burst open a floodgate of tears, now surging down my cheeks with unstoppable force.

Andrew had expressed many times before that leaving tea rings on the counter pushed his buttons. When I look back now, maybe my action of leaving the tea ring had simply been a covert act of my subconscious, knowing what buttons to push to create personal space. Was I sabotaging our relationship in order to close the door on him—and the world?

Would this new challenge make or break our relationship? I wondered, realizing that circumstances in my surroundings had the potential to hinder or promote my recovery. Fearing that I had too much at stake, I wasn't prepared to take any chances.

Over the next few days I worked on getting my head around the list of professionals for my doctor. As I had been a creative director for many years, it was only fitting that I would approach this task as if gathering the team for my next project. From my experience, I knew that the success of large projects depended on synergy being created, the glue that ties the whole project together.

Little did I know, but I had experienced synergy when I had faced Goliath before—when a group of total strangers appeared from nowhere to help raise awareness about the issues faced by peanut allergic passengers. I didn't know these people, and even though I am eternally grateful that they came forward, together we conquered a common goal.

I had a new Goliath and knew instinctively what I needed to do—to gather a group of people to work as a whole on my recovery project rather than have them working separately. I needed to join the dots—not to scatter them. Therefore, I approached my doctor's request as I would a creative project and made the following outline:

My Project

Purpose
To remove the threat of cancer; to restore mental, physical, and emotional well-being

Approach
Utilize synergy to create a supportive environment to promote recovery and healing

Deadline
180 days

Requirements
To maintain safety at all costs
100% commitment to my health and well-being
Love and caring, empathy and understanding, and openness

Policies and Procedures
Allergy Management and Emergency Action Plan

Factors of Influence
Space
Time
Money
Other people
Emotional stability: frequent arguments, sensitivity to criticism, walking on egg shells, unable to write journals on a deep level for fear they will be found and used against me, low self-esteem, and unresolved trauma all must be resolved. Uncertainty must be addressed
Control
Diet
Knowledge

My Team

Director and Project Coordinator
Me

Team Leader
My doctor

To liaise between specialists and professionals; to write prescriptions and referral letters when required; to spend time explaining results such as blood tests, x-rays, ultrasounds, scans, etc, and how my body will work to heal itself

Specialist (s)
To offer expertise and knowledge on their particular field of study or specialty

Provisional list
Nutritionist/Dietician on food and nutrition
Physiotherapist on physical body
Psychologist on emotional and mental health
Somatic psychotherapy, and so on

Spokesperson
My health situation becomes the dominant and only topic of conversation especially when talking about illness, and this unknowingly trains the subconscious mind to support the manifestation of the condition. Nominate a friend to tell others about my progress. That way I will only have to speak to one person about it

Historians/source of childhood history
My family

Resources and tools
o Medical history, test results, records of hospital admissions, and treatment
o Leaflets, brochures, or information cards to explain the problem to others
o Diary/Journal
o Lockable cashbox to hold my journal from uninvited eyes

Evaluating project success
Medical tests showing negative results (in medical terms, a negative result indicates the absence of the disease or condition for which the test was made)
Space to breathe
Peace and to feel grounded

Now I had a plan. For the first time in relation to my own health, I had created a positive goal to propel myself towards. I had clarity and direction to focus my attention, and I had the makings of the team to help me get there.

My Goal

That in 180 days, test results show that the threat of cancer is gone, well-being is restored, and I have space to breathe at peace on my own solid ground. Only time would tell if this exercise had simply been a desperate clinging to the little hope I had left, or if it was the start of something more. I'll let you decide.

Over the next 180 days, the following chain of events took place:

o I delivered the list of professionals to my doctor
o I was placed on an Australian Government health care plan available to patients that have a chronic condition and complex care needs being managed by their GP
o A team of specialists was gathered. This opened a new line of support, and access to specific knowledge and care
o My family rallied together to raise thousands of dollars required for my operation
o A dietician helped me to design a new eating plan by my specific request
o I had an operation to cut out the cancer cell anomalies. An allergic reaction to the treatment followed
o By now I was seeing a psychologist in the evening once a week. Her main area of expertise was in helping victims of trauma
o Andrew continued to look for work for me
o The funds were raised to travel to Europe where I'd return to Germany for the first time after a decade
o I would go to the site of the sexual assault and raise a glass of champagne with a couple of friends in celebration, knowing that this chapter in my life had been finally put to rest
o Upon my return to Sydney, tests revealed that the threat of cancer was no more
o I learned that I had another "incurable" to deal with when Graves disease, an autoimmune disease of my thyroid gland, was diagnosed

- o I adapted my project to include this new burden, knowing that it was the remainder of unresolved trauma trapped in another part of my body
- o I started visits to an endocrinologist (a specialist of the glands)
- o Like *déjà vu* I was told that there was a strong probability I was allergic to the normal treatment for Graves Disease, suggesting an operation. This time I chose not to go ahead with it, to follow my own path
- o My blood was analyzed by a series of blood tests every three weeks. This gave me a way to measure the progress of my healing project
- o I began to see a physiotherapist three times a week. We worked together on releasing pain trapped deep within my body. She introduced me to Ortho-Bionomy®.
- o Andrew and I broke up
- o My family helped me to gather the funds together to purchase my first property
- o I moved into my own home, which was close to my friends, soon finding a job in my profession with a boss who was empathetic to my specific needs
- o Medical tests revealed that Graves Disease was no more
- o There was a new sense of peace in my soul

Following the break-up with Andrew, every so often we would meet to catch up on how we were both doing. On one occasion we spoke about the ring of tea on the counter. I had come to recognize that, even though his response to the shocking news that day had seemed harsh and uncaring, it was as perfect as it could have been. I genuinely thanked him for it. Would I be where I am now if he had reacted any differently? Probably not! His reaction was an impetus to me taking responsibility for my own health on every level.

I truly did have plenty to thank him for.

11

What We Resist or Submit to Persists
"Life isn't about finding yourself.
Life is about creating yourself."
Unknown

One day I finally realized why my allergies couldn't possibly have been resolved before that moment.

I had the kind of frustration flowing through my blood that makes you want to be a baby, yelling and waving your fists about. I was unable to put into words the bitterness that was oozing from the essence of my being. The world, society, medicine, and my body had forsaken me. They had let me down again to make sense of all my health problems alone. My life seemed to be a failure on all levels.

Five months had passed since the day at the doctor's office. I was eternally grateful to the people who had come together to help me, and more so that the threat of cancer was now a thing of the past. So was Grave's disease, an autoimmune disease of the thyroid gland, that had been discovered a mere three months after my cancer diagnosis.

It had become evident that a chain of events had been necessary to lead me to this point. Both health challenges were different, yet the end result was the same—a solution was found. Despite not following in any sequence or order, the essence of each challenge and approach had striking resemblances.

I had created a supportive environment to promote healing, had increased my level of health intelligence to clearly identify the problem, I had adapted proven strategies to suit my particular circumstances, I had incorporated the new learning into my lifestyle, and I had let go of unnecessary baggage to create space for my body to heal. In the whole experience I had tapped into and witnessed the power of an innate inner intelligence. I didn't heal myself; rather the innate health intelligence did all that for me. Instead of thinking that healing was just about going through a mind over body experience, I now knew that it was quite the opposite. I had learned to TRUST guidance from within, and follow step by step processes such as adjusting my diet or whatever was necessary to remove the problem once it revealed itself. Now, even though I was humbled by the amazing healing journey I had undergone so far, I still felt wounded. My allergies were still very much alive and well, and I still felt indescribable amounts of anger surging within.

How could this powerful inner intelligence get rid of a health problem that had shadowed my whole life? I thought this, feeling rage energizing every cell in my body as I glanced at my allergy test results to date. Had my sensitivity levels become too much for this innate wisdom to handle? Recalling the multitude of self-help and inspirational books I had read about survivors of cancer and other miraculous healings, I was trying to believe. My quest for knowledge had become an obsession, fine tuned to receive only the information about the particular health challenge I was facing at the time. At least this time my obsession focused on delivering something positive— steps towards healing rather than how to just get on with life.

Each source spoke about getting in touch with a powerful innate intelligence, which from the time of our conception steers our lives through bodily sensations, feelings, thoughts, and even dreams. The sources said that every experience we have throughout our lifetimes is registered in the body; the memory is imprinted in our cells and in our consciousness.

Why was this inner intelligence unable to circumvent my allergies— especially when it had access to all there was to know about me? Puzzled by this, I couldn't help but think of my dear friend Fritz. How fortunate I was that he came into my life when he did, recalling the question he asked me when I first told him about my allergies.

In fact, I informed every potential friend at first introduction that I was allergic to peanuts. Being up front about the risks meant that I could get that part out of the way. It also gave them the opportunity to ask questions, politely reject me, or pass judgment before any harm was done; before either of us could start to care.

Like clockwork on a Friday night, I'd go to the local club to meet friends and share stories about the week. A year had passed since I had first arrived in Sydney, and I was such a regular at the club, they had set up a peanut-free zone for me. Despite the "zone" being a very small area in the corner of the main lounge, I was delighted with it. It was my oasis: a place to relax with peace of mind and talk to my heart's content with newfound friends.

Fritz, an ex-pat from Germany, first entered my life in 1997. Only now do I recognize the significance of our meeting as the first step on my path to unfolding. He had moved to Australia only a few years before and was a certified re-birthing practitioner well-versed in personal development. He worked at Sydney airport assisting special needs passengers.

As usual, my allergies came up in conversation. Fritz listened intently as I gave him the well-rehearsed allergy spiel, laughing when I told him about the incident during the blizzard in Washington. It didn't take long before my laughter was dissolved in indignation.

"Why did you create your allergies?" he asked in an inquisitive tone as he lifted his beer glass to take a drink.

I had just explained the ins and outs of my peanut allergy to him and couldn't believe his question.

Did I hear him right? I asked myself. Is he blaming me? I couldn't believe my ears.

"Why in the world do you think I caused something like this? My allergies were there long before I found out they existed. It's not my fault I have this," I replied, feeling tension build in my muscles as I took a defensive stance.

"Well…" he replied, but I immediately cut in before he could continue. I wasn't interested in hearing what he had to say.

"It's just the card that life has dealt me. It's as simple as that. I just have to learn to live with it. That's it in a nutshell," I said, obviously annoyed.

The thought that he was blaming me for creating such a volatile deadly reaction pissed me off. I was also too terrified to even ponder on his question for fear of what I might discover if I ever did attempt to answer it.

"If you created the allergies, then they can be uncreated," he continued.

"Please stop! I told you already…nothing can be done about them…even my doctors agree with me…end of story."

"But I am curious to know your answer," he retorted.

"Please...I don't need you, or anyone else for that matter, becoming an allergy removal expert all of a sudden," I exclaimed, clearly displaying contempt in my hardened posture.

I wasn't prepared even to consider his point of view.

"I'll be back in a minute," I muttered under my breath, departing from my oasis. I was disgusted by his lack of empathy upon hearing my plight, unwilling to waste any more of my breath on him as I made a beeline to the bathroom.

They can be uncreated. Huh! What rubbish!

Anyway, if I could uncreate my allergies from my life, what would I do? How would I cope? They were me—my life. My allergies defined my existence; they were entwined in the very fabric of my being. They were the core of the person I had come to be. I wasn't willing to let go of the only life I knew so well, and I would kick and scream with all my might if anyone tried to take that from me.

So much so, that if anyone ever claimed to be able to remove my allergies, they would feel my wrath. It would be like trying to steal a soul from heaven; there would be absolutely no way they could conquer the wrath of God to follow. The fortress of my will, which had taken a lifetime to build, was too strong to penetrate.

Deep down, I knew Fritz had only been trying to help me, and I reacted as if he was attempting to murder my best friend. Why was I defending my allergies? If a real friend brought so much heartache and trauma into my life, they would automatically get their marching papers. Did I simply give power to my allergies because I believed I couldn't do anything about them? Or did I want them in some way?

Why had I been the loyal defender of the source of so much turmoil? What possible benefit was there to hanging onto them? There had to be something that I was not willing to look at. I would come to realize this much later, but I had a few more life lessons to learn first.

Over the next few years, Fritz and I became really good friends. Given our first encounter, I jokingly introduced him as my "spiritual advisor" to newcomers to our group. Over time, his spirit shone like a bright beacon in my darkest hours. He held my hand through the most unforgiving challenges, and he sparked my interest in personal development and my own consciousness.

My life had followed a series of downward spirals and was about to reach rock bottom. I had tried everything to keep my head above water, but nothing seemed to be working. The mask of deception that everything was okay had begun to crack.

I had been drowning in a sea of alcohol in hope of sweeping the anguish away, when in the eleventh hour to total breakdown, I surrendered. The walls of the great fortress crumbled around me, and a doorway opened to the path of change. For the first time in my life, I reached out for help.

I turned to my dear friend Fritz. We had been on a safari through South Africa's wilderness, we had climbed castles in Ireland, but he really came into my life as the gatekeeper to a path that would lead me far beyond my wildest dreams.

My interest in personal development and consciousness began to flourish. I took an introductory weekend course that was fittingly called "The Turning Point". This course would lead to ongoing studies about what made me tick. I continue these studies to date. Some of the topics included childhood development, conflict resolution, stress and health management, bioenergetics (the subject of a field of biochemistry that concerns energy flow through living systems), somatic therapy (recognition and release of energy stored in the body), emotional intelligence, belief systems, and the evolution of consciousness. I became a wealth of knowledge, understanding more about myself and my life than ever before. Yet no matter how many books I read or personal development courses I took, one thing always stood its ground—my allergy.

Today, by trusting my inner wisdom to guide me back in time, I finally realize why my allergies could never be resolved before. Giving in to the belief that there is no cure for Anaphylaxis prevented me from even trying to look for a solution. Up to that point, I never once went beyond looking for solutions for my day-to-day challenges, or even thought it possible to be able to delve deep within to find out what was really going on. But that was about to change.

Initially I was skeptical when I heard about the innate inner wisdom inside all of us. Now I can see the results for myself. My healing journey so far has given me newfound hope and confidence as well as the courage to delve deeper into finding the source of all this suffering.

I wasn't born with allergies; they manifested later. So maybe there was some truth after all to the notion that something in me had created this condition in my life. I finally got the lesson that Fritz had entered my life to teach me and became living proof that it is possible to create—and recreate—yourself.

There just might be a chance I can resolve my allergies, I thought, as a rush of confidence and hope flowed through my veins like never before. It is time to take responsibility for your own allergy healing, said a powerful voice inside my head

Resistance to delve deep inside instantly dissolved, unlocking the pathway to the cause of my reaction.

For the first time in my life I actually realized that I was the creator of my own health situation. I saw that the next step was to shine a light on the presenting problem to see it with fresh eyes in order to identify exactly what I was dealing with. I knew that once I knew more about the problem then I would be in a better position to find a solution.

Understanding the next step on my journey, I turned to my inner wisdom for guidance.

12

Meeting with a VIP

"A mentor is someone who allows you to see the hope inside yourself."
Oprah Winfrey

"It is time to face my allergies," I thought. I now knew beyond a shadow of a doubt that I could beat this enemy once and for all. I had mobilized my resources against the threat of cancer, and I had new resources to boot. Yet, since Anaphylaxis had never been conquered before, I knew that to figure out a solution I had to look in unknown, unexplored territory beyond the normal way of thinking. My burning questions needed answers, but there just didn't seem to be enough hours in my day to explore it. It was like trying to make time to learn a new language. Who could readily take that on?

"How am I ever going to have the time to figure this out?" I thought, thinking of my busy schedule. I was already working from dawn till dusk in a new job; I had all the usual adult responsibilities, plus it took almost forever in the supermarket to read labels, and I cooked everything from scratch. My list of doctor and specialist appointments seemed almost endless, and any spare time was booked solid with meeting with friends—a support system no one can really do without.

I was struggling to find time for myself. At the same time, I knew that if I was not 100% committed to my health and recovery, I could easily let the healing process slide or make up an excuse to do something else when times got tough. This time I was determined to keep going, to endure, and to stay committed. My life depended on it. In fact, by this stage my life depended on almost everything I did. It was crucial to prioritize my schedule. I had to make friends with time again rather than complain that it was always slipping away and was uncontrollable.

Then I thought of Oprah. I had been fortunate enough to have watched her show live from the audience when I lived in Chicago in 1991. She was a source of inspiration and role model in my life. If I was ever so lucky as to have an hour with her in person, I would do absolutely everything in my power to make sure the appointment went ahead. Nothing would stop me. The opportunity to learn from her wisdom and experience would be too important to miss.

I reasoned, "My life, health, and wellbeing are just as, if not more, important than a meeting with Oprah, right?" I thought. "Then what is stopping me from making a VIP appointment with the most important person in my world—me?

Absolutely nothing!"

Over the next few weeks I incorporated five minutes of VIP "me" time into every waking hour of my day. I allocated VIP time to scan inward, to give all my undivided attention to listen to what was going on inside. It's very different from taking time out to watch TV, catch up with friends, or go to a game. If Oprah ever came to my house for a visit, do you think I would spend my precious time with her watching TV? Definitely not! I would give my guest all my undivided attention in order to listen and learn from the experience, and that's what I began to give myself during my VIP time.

For example, during my VIP time I'd scan my body for any build up of stress or muscle tension, check in with how I was feeling, and monitor my thoughts for any negativity. If any muscle tension was found, a simple stretch at my desk at work released it; if I was feeling unstable or had scattered thoughts, I'd take a moment to close my eyes and visualize my feet firmly rooted in the ground.

The new diagnosis in the doctor's office was a "gift", as I had begun to listen to the symptoms and signs from my body's innate internal messaging system.

This simple task of scanning and releasing went unnoticed by others, yet it made a huge impact on my general state of mind, my emotions, and physical well-being. Within a few weeks, the results were dramatic. My body was under less pressure from daily stresses and tension, my thoughts had more clarity, and I had more control over my emotions, feeling a sense of stability and grounding. I became more productive in my day-to-day activities as my mind and body knew they were being taken care of and listened to.

I had a better perspective on what was really going on inside of me. Listening to my body's internal messaging system gave me clarity and direction, and it set a firm foundation for a path to recovery and healing. Even though I still had to remain vigilant to prevent an allergic reaction, and I also had other responsibilities to uphold, constantly removing the daily build-up of stress meant that more time and energy were freed up to focus on deeper level issues engrained over a longer period of time.

Gradually, my five minutes of VIP time every hour was extended by adding a one hour block of VIP time at the end of each day. This was to incorporate longer release strategies such as meditation to clear the mind, further research if required, journal writing, or to perform a particular exercise which required a different setting and/or more time to release a specific block.

Eventually, I'd add a VIP pamper day per month.

One day, the first Saturday of the month of September, was a VIP pampering day. I awoke on this day with many questions on my lips. I had come to recognize that manifestations of symptoms or disease are messages or signals from within—designed to let the person know when something isn't working as efficiently as it should and that conscious intervention is required.

"If my mind could have figured the source of my problem out, it would have done so a long time ago," I thought. This told me that the answer I sought resided some place deeper than the mind. To access it required the right setting, removed from the hustle and bustle and distractions of daily life.

The early days of spring in Sydney have always been my favorite time of the year. It is when the winter, which I fondly call an Irish summer, draws to a close. The temperature is not too hot and not too cold. It is similar to the median Irish climate I was used to.

Spring is a time that represents renewal, rejuvenation, recharge, new beginnings, and waking from hibernation after a long, barren winter. It was my time to wake up, to delve deep and to start a new journey to another beginning. One significant new beginning in my life sprung to mind. It was when I was about eight years old, we moved to a new family home on the outskirts of Dublin. The house is situated at a crossroads, in the midst of rolling fields, apple orchards, and dairy farms, all connected by a small river, which is the vein of the community. It is close to a reservoir, which was the home of lifelong partners—a pair of white swans. On top of a hill, a small church overlooks an oasis bursting with natural beauty. The birds' unique lullabies can be heard for miles, squirrels and hedgehogs are plentiful, rabbits run wild, horses and cows graze on the vibrant green grass, and ruins of old castles and hillside graveyards whisper stories of the past in the wind.

It was a magical and spiritual place for a child growing up, full of folklore, superstition, tradition, or local tales of the latest haunting. I often wonder if the whispered ghost stories were designed to scare the local children from trespassing, or if the history of the surroundings actually had a message to tell its inhabitants. All in all, the idea that ghosts might be among us fascinated me. I always had my ear to the ground, looking for a sign that they existed. Their existence might explain some of the things that I couldn't. I was forever in hope that they would give me a sign.

When trying to make some sense of the world as a teenager, I'd go for a walk to the end of our road to a small picturesque stone bridge erected over the river. There I'd find a comfortable place to sit on the luscious grass by the waterside to gather my thoughts or write in my diary. Being next to water and surrounded by nature always gave me comfort when my mind was troubled or when I needed to replenish.

"Go to the water and I will be there."

I can still recall the words my great grandmother said to me the last time I saw her alive. Even though she passed when I was in my twenties, her message only reinforced where to go when I needed comfort and guidance. Therefore, on this VIP day at that time of year, I decided to follow my great grandmother's advice and go to a place in nature beside the water, taking with me only my personal journal and my favorite purple pen.

Centennial Park is a large public, urban park that occupies 220 hectares in the eastern suburbs of Sydney. It could provide me with all the elements needed to recreate the settings wherein I could access forgotten memories of the past. The park has wide open spaces of green fields, horses, historical monuments next to pine and native forests, and vast areas of water with ornamental lakes, which are home to many swans and ducks.

My most cherished place was the center of the park, where a small white bridge passed over water next to my favorite old tree. This spot overlooked swampland and forest areas and offered shade as protection from the glaring Australian sun. Passers-by were minimal; the sounds of the city were nothing more than a distant hum, and the flora and fauna were plentiful.

Sitting under the tree on a bright red and green checkered rug, I began to write. This type of writing was different than what I had learned at school. I used a writing technique I read about in self help books and learned at personal development courses, which I adapted to my circumstances and later dubbed as "Intuitive Writing".

First, I'd create a list of questions that I wanted to ask my infinite higher intelligence. Then I would create the optimum setting, and then with my *non-dominant* hand, I would write down thoughts, feelings, bodily sensations, ideas, insights, or anything else that sprung to mind. To my surprise, this type of writing helped me to access unknown, unexplored territories of my mind and body; to get past layers of muck created over time; and to plummet deep into my subconscious to access to a wealth of stuff I didn't consciously know or remember.

As the pen touched the paper, one small speck of dust on the ground caught my eye as it glistened in the sun. Millions of grains surrounding it rested under my feet, yet this one shone brightly in its glory, reflecting the rays of the sun. The more I focused on this one grain of light, the more I saw others just like it. It was when I paid some attention to the surrounding area that I noticed many other specks glistening around me. Each speck was an individual and yet part of the same ground. When the sun moved across the sky, all the specks took their turns shining.

That's interesting! I thought. The closer I look at something, the more it reveals itself. I was pondering this as I switched the pen to my non-dominant hand to start "Intuitive Writing". I began to scribble a whole load of questions down on paper, acknowledging that my subconscious mind knew the answers to them all.

What is it about peanuts that cause an allergic reaction? What exactly is Anaphylaxis? How can I move forward when I'm afraid to make a mistake? A part of me wants to let go of this problem, but another part doesn't. What do I do? Where do I start when I'm already struggling to keep up?

From all the books I had read, I had learned that once the subconscious mind accepts an idea, it begins to execute it straight away. It follows one law, and that is to work toward the ideas it is given, whether they are good or bad ideas, like a self-fulfilling prophecy. You know when the subconscious truly speaks, as the words are the clearest, it always tells the truth, and it contains only love. Anything less comes from somewhere else and is therefore false.

The subconscious does not know it knows unless asked, it will not talk back, argue or judge; it is obedient, and works 24/7 behind the scenes to fulfill what you want it to. In relation to the powerful instrument that is the subconscious, the old Chinese saying becomes transparently true: "Be careful what you wish for—you may get it!" Yet how many of us take the time to tap into this powerful source and resource to find our way on our paths in life?

Thoughts and ideas began to bubble to the surface, and as if an invisible force took a hold of my pen, it started to write on its own...the VIP meeting with my infinite inner intelligence had begun, and I was extremely interested in what it might have to say.

13

Uncut Words of Wisdom

"Write down the thoughts of the moment.
Those that come unsought for are commonly
the most valuable."

Francis Bacon

The following excerpts come from my personal journals written over a five year period. Not only did these words answer some of my questions, they also acted as signposts on my path to healing. Even though everyone's path to healing is unique, I have listed the words of wisdom which pertain to the rest of my journey as told in this book.

☜∘☞

You unconsciously react to stimuli in your internal and external environments every second of the day, even when you sleep. The type of reaction and its outcome has a fundamental impact on everything in your life. It can influence the way you behave or don't, what you believe, your mood, your attitudes, cravings or addictions, wellness or disease, your surroundings and the people in it, your spirituality, and ultimately who you are.

☜∘☞

Your reactions are dictated by how nature has shaped you and by what you have learned from experience. They are tied to triggers that can be changed.

☜∘☞

Where a reaction fires off or activates determines the outcome. Understanding the anatomy of unwanted reactions gives you power to change to a desired outcome.

☜∘☞

The allergen is not the problem; it is how the body reacts to it that is the problem.

❧❧

Many questions asked about illness look to the effect's side of the problem for an answer. But the answers you seek reside at the source or causal side. Like a speck of dust, each symptom or end result appears in response to a shift in the surrounding environment or particular set of circumstances. Yet only when it appears do you notice, eventually believing that the condition itself is actually the cause of your upset, rather than it simply being the results or effects from cause.

❧❧

Take a look at the side of healing that you are most familiar with—the place where the majority of the world resides. It is a system of diagnosis and treatment based on science that starts with causes. In truth, a group of abnormal signs and symptoms are the effects of or reactions to a cause. Most traditional medicine relies on dealing with the effects or symptoms, ignoring the cause.

A surgeon removes a growth; a growth which cannot possibly have come into existence without a cause. It grew in response to a cause and has a strong likelihood of coming back again because the cause is left untouched. This can be seen in some cancer cases where problem cells are surgically removed yet return somewhere else in the body months or even years later. The underlying cause that mutated the healthy cells in the first place was ignored.

❧❧

Do you think for one minute your body would create such a violent reaction to something otherwise harmless without having a due cause? First, there must be a change in the condition of the body's fluids and tissues to give rise to a systemic impairment or lowered resistance. A reaction cannot possibly come into existence without a cause. Look to the cause to change the reaction.

❧❧

There is a multitude of drugs on the market to treat every physical or mental symptom imaginable. If it comes in a bottle and it can be sold, then it's guaranteed to become mainstream.

We have become accustomed to taking pills as a quick fix in the hope they will remove the pain of disease. These drugs only temporarily mask the symptoms, which may show up later in life as another symptom or condition until the cause is addressed.

ودو

A reaction sits on the "effects" side of the equation. Stay in action and there resides "cause".

ودو

Imagine the human body is split into two parts: Half is chemistry and the other half is physics. Traditional medicine is only concerned with chemistry, and it ignores physics. Much of human health is influenced by physics.

Physics cannot be bottled and sold like chemistry is; hence, it is ignored. This is probably why scientists struggle to find a wonder drug to fix all ailments. They see only half of the picture.

ودو

Today science is so advanced yet new generations of scientists must, without any doubt trust that the doctors and scientists of yesteryear got the foundations right the first time. They know that to repeat earlier work in today's age would cost a great deal. They have also learned the stereotyped treatment that comes with each ailment; anti-histamines for colds and allergies; an operation for cell anomalies; morphine for cancer; and so on. Once the official naming ceremony is over, rarely do we look beyond the name or associated treatment to find, understand or eliminate the cause.

ودو

Everything you see, eat, smell, hear, think, dream, touch, and feel on a daily basis is connected to you on a cellular level—as to your blood. Allergies and other health disorders are in the blood. Look closer there, and you will find some answers.

ودو

Scientific research shows that while measuring the frequencies in the human body, there is a distinct difference between healthy and unhealthy ones. Illness, infection, or disease can only exist at particular frequencies. It's these waves of energy that vibrate areas of our brain and body. Our nerves send the messages to our brain and body about the vibration. The vibration is then interpreted as sight, sound, smell, taste, touch, or as an emotion. The action of the different waves and vibrations moving around in our minds and bodies cause the area to respond according to the frequency passing through it.

❧

Most of what our bodies learn as children, we pick up from mimicking others or from our surroundings. Sometimes the body can get it wrong or make a mistake from the information it has received and/or mimicked. Go back to basics and learn again.

❧

Anxiety, stubbornness, fear, anger, blame, and other negative emotions are more than just feelings or sensations in the body. Look to the science behind emotions, as they can be measured.

❧

Your particular body structure and how you hold yourself has a tendency to dictate how you react to situations or circumstances.

❧

The food you eat has its own frequency, vibration, energy, and life force, which you cannot see but you can feel. The energy extracted from food is attracted to the area in the body that functions at the same frequency. Bodily functions running at abnormal frequencies than normal are more susceptible to malfunction or harm from displaced energy. This is why some food is good for certain bodily parts and damaging to others.

❧

We are all born with a gift, and that is to heal. We all have an amazingly complex body, made up of approximately 75 to 100 trillion cells (adult body), that regenerate on a regular basis. Scientific evidence shows that we have a new body every couple of years with parts that are much younger than all of our birthdays.

୬⊶ଔ

I come with many names. To some, I am known as the healer, teacher, mentor, or guide, and to others, a gift, higher intelligence, inner wisdom, consciousness, authentic self, higher being, human spirit, soul, or light. I am in every cell of your body and all around you, the space between the space, inside and outside of you. You cannot see me, but I am always here. I speak to you all the time. In fact, I work for you all the time, making sure that everything in your body and mind are functioning at their optimum.

When you cut yourself, I create new skin where the old layer has been lost; I knit together a bone when it is fractured; I tell you to eat when your stomach is empty; I regenerate and repair damage to your cells; and I send you messages to warn you of an imbalance in your body, or when you are in danger of losing your health.

୬⊶ଔ

Internal chatter is nothing more than mere utterances or noise, trying to convince you that the obstacles to your goals are insurmountable. Take heed, as words are the least effective communicator. They are most often misunderstood, misinterpreted, or come from others. Most often this voice serves only to confuse or stop you from moving forward. The difficulty comes in telling the difference between these utterances and what *I* say. You know my words. They are the clearest, they always tell the truth, and they contain only love. Anything less comes from another source and is therefore false.

୬⊶ଔ

The human mind works better if it moves towards what it wants rather than what it doesn't.

୬⊶ଔ

The physical brain is a function of your thoughts. You can change your brain structure by what you think. Your body is a function of your feelings.

୬⊶ଔ

Everybody believes that they have a good memory. This isn't true. Every time something is remembered or recalled, the biochemistry of the brain changes. This means that memories can be altered, easily distorted, and faulty.

᷼

As children we learn that the mind is separate.

᷼

The body always tells the truth. Learn to listen.

᷼

You are in total control of your own conversation. At the end of the day you are the only one to make the decision about how you want it to be. When you are willing to hear my message, you become more open to receiving it, to call it your own, and to act on it.

᷼

The result of you not listening is that you will keep re-living the same problem over and over again until you eventually heed my message and do something about it.

Judgment is often based on an attachment to a past experience. When judgment appears in conversation, the openness to hear the message is automatically shut out or blocked. Then you either resist or submit. What you resist or submit to will persist.

᷼

You endlessly receive messages from me through your thoughts, feelings, experiences, and physical symptoms. A physical message may start out as a discomfort, and when I don't get your attention, I yell at you by turning it into a pain, a dream into a nightmare, a sensitivity into an allergy, and so on. When all efforts still fail to get your attention to act, I have to scream at you, manifesting into disease, hardship, mental illness, and so on.

You already know what happens when you do not heed my messages. That is why when diagnosis comes, it is a blessing or wake up call to hear my message and to begin a conversation.

᷼

Most people looking to heal themselves instinctively move into survival mode. In doing so, the disease or illness also gets the message to survive. A battle begins. Accessing the gap between healing and cell regeneration is where you need to go. The space between the space is where you will find me.

৵৽৽

Scientific research shows that our mind speaks directly to our immune system and emotions. We can talk directly to our mind through our thoughts. Therefore, it is possible to speak directly to our immune system through our mind and emotions.

৵৽৽

When the immune system is strong enough to do its job properly, the odds are that you are healthy. When it stumbles, foreign agents including bacteria, viruses, parasites, fungi, and even disease can gain a foothold inside you.

৵৽৽

An overactive immune system needs to find peace, not more strength to fight.

৵৽৽

Attempting to deceive or desensitize the mind, body, immune system, or emotions is like masking a ticking bomb that is just waiting for the right moment to go off.

৵৽৽

Take a closer look at the presenting problem and your pathway to healing will reveal itself. The physical symptoms, behavior, thoughts, emotions, end result, or other responses associated with the problem are blessings. They are the signposts on your pathway of discovery to a solution, cause, source, and maybe even a cure. Signposts give you a place to start and a holistic view of the presenting problem.

৵৽৽

14

Peanut Allergy Is on the Rise—But What Does This Tell Us?

"The answer you seek is in the question you ask."
Journal Extract: Michelle Flanagan

I had so many questions about my peanut allergy. Every question I asked seemed to open up another line of questions to explore. But to get the necessary answers for my path of unfoldment, it was important that I looked at what I already knew with fresh eyes and asked the right questions. This would take my journey of discovery back to my childhood world and even further.

Following an extreme allergic incident a few months after I first arrived in Sydney, I had become a serial hunter and gatherer of information. My home was filled with endless boxes full of newspaper clippings, videos or anything else I could find about my main enemy—the peanut. Family and friends added to this collection from time to time, and I was holding onto absolutely everything. If it might one day shed some new light on my plight, it was stored or hoarded. Over the years it had become a personal mission to find answers. I had become disheartened that my questions delivered no results. But I persevered regardless, keeping every little piece of whatever meaningful cast-off bit of information that might one day become the missing pieces to my great puzzle, my work in progress.

I likewise kept a list of questions. Why, for example, was I allergic but my sister and brother weren't? We had the same parents. Mum didn't eat peanuts when pregnant with any of us. We were raised alike, had the same vaccinations, and we ate the same simple food in childhood. Why, then, was I the only one in my family to develop the worst form of allergy known? And why an allergy to peanuts as opposed to any other food? There had to be something from my childhood I had overlooked.

What had been going on in my early years? On my path of unfoldment I was drawn to ask these same questions I'd asked for years but this time I was armed with increased health intelligence as well as guidance from within. What could the history of this particular food tell me now that might shed a new light or show me something I hadn't recognized before?

The history of the peanut told me that only a decade before my birth peanuts were first introduced as snacks in bars, thus dubbing the packaged product "Beer Nuts". Peanuts were promoted to bar owners as a snack that would sell more beer, and they spread like wildfire. By 1969, the year I was born, ten million pounds of the nuts were produced a year for bars in the United States alone. Bars and clubs had now become a popular place for both men and women to meet. This was a far cry from ten years before, when bars were places only men frequented. Now both sexes increased consumption of bagged peanuts as a healthy and readily available snack.

The early '60s also saw the introduction of the oral contraceptive pill, prescribed only to married women until 1967. The drug worked by giving the body an extra boost of hormones (synthetic estrogen and synthetic progesterone in the first Pill), to prevent pregnancy. Women could now focus on their careers. They had more buying power and control over their fertility.

Birth rates were tapering, as were the number of breast feeding mothers at home. By the end of the '60s, approximately 75% of American babies were fed commercially produced baby formulas in their first year. In Ireland, on the other side of the Atlantic, I too was fed baby formula as opposed to being breastfed. I do not make any connections between peanuts and the oral contraceptive pill but simply say this to show widespread changes in Western society at the time.

By the '70s, the peanut had become a national icon in the United States. It was heavily marketed to children as a healthy, inexpensive snack through children's books, cookbooks, toys, songs, and cartoon characters. The first children's peanut cookbook was published in 1976 by Natalie Donna, author of *Peanut Craft*. Let's not forget the decades-running, wildly popular comic strip with the title *Peanuts*, or that fact that President Jimmy Carter was a peanut farmer!

Some of their popularity may be ascribed to the fact that peanuts appear to be healthy. According to nutritionists, peanuts are an excellent source of protein, and they contain vitamin B-12, vitamin E, magnesium, chromium, and manganese. These are nutrients typically found in meats, whole grains, legumes, and vegetable oils, yet peanuts were an inexpensive source.

The peanut industry, understandably, was flourishing—so much so that there was little or no research in the field of peanut allergy until later. How could this rich source of protein be seen as anything but harmless and healthy?

Asthma was the childhood health concern of the time, another serious and debilitating form of allergy. It was reported in England and Wales that hospital admission rates for childhood asthma increased substantially during the 1960s (rates trebled among newborns to four-year-olds from 1962 to 1969 and doubled among five to fourteen-year-olds), and continued to increase throughout the 1970s and early 1980s.

Before the development of the RAST allergy test in 1972, allergic symptoms often went unrecognized and incorrect treatment was given. Allergic reactions simply weren't attributed to a snack so good for you so doctors recommended it as a highly nutritious and inexpensive source of easily digestible protein to pregnant and breastfeeding women. All that changed in the '90s when newspaper articles with new findings began to emerge. Somehow, this advice from doctors given over a twenty year period was retracted, and science turned the focus on pregnant mums and their diet as possible cause of peanut allergy in children.

"Pregnant mothers could be sensitizing their unborn children by eating peanut-based foods," an article in a UK newspaper reported in 1995. Everyone wanted to know why the number of children with peanut allergy was growing rapidly:

"Peanut allergy now affects one in 80 children under five; that's approximately 50,000 pre-school-age children at risk," reported research by The Asthma and Allergy Research Centre, also in 1995.

Although pregnant women were now advised to avoid eating peanuts, the numbers of children diagnosed with peanut allergy still continued to rise. Another study conducted in 1998 was not conclusive that diet during pregnancy led to this allergy.

I asked my mum if she ate peanuts during pregnancy when carrying me. She said, "Definitely not."

In 2009, Australian research found that peanut avoidance during pregnancy and in the early years was counterproductive. Yet, contrary to their findings, a study in the November 1, 2010 issue of the *Journal of Allergy and Clinical Immunology* found that allergic infants might be at increased risk of peanut allergy if their mothers ingested peanuts during pregnancy. There seemed to be too many conflicting reports, achieving very little except to point blame in some direction or another. Unfortunately, in the line of fire are the mums, who are usually just trying to do their best for themselves and their children.

My dad was sensitive to peanuts. He would get a sore throat if he ate them, and therefore they weren't on my family's menu. My mum didn't particularly like the taste of peanuts, so they weren't in my environment when my mum was pregnant with me or in my infancy. Then what could have caused my body to react in such a way? Had Dad simply transferred his sensitivity on to me through his genes? But why was I the only allergic one in the family? In fact, I was the only one on both sides of my family with peanut Anaphylaxis. And my extended family, a long line of blood relatives, is large. This life threatening condition just seemed to materialize from nowhere. But I knew this wasn't true. I wasn't born that way. My allergies came later. What had changed since my birth?

If peanut avoidance is counterproductive, then what other factors might influence a child's physical and mental development to manifest this? After all, children are like sponges, subconsciously absorbing all the information around them. Their minds and bodies are still young, taking in and processing what they don't yet fully understand.

Or could there have been something in the food, or water maybe? India and China have peanuts and/or other nuts as part of their main diet. Pregnant women and young infants in both of these countries eat peanuts on a regular basis. Yet statistics show that the prevalence of peanut allergy cases in both these two countries is the lowest worldwide. Was there something in their culture that was different from the West? Vaccinations? Baby formula? Or even the way they prepared and cooked peanuts? But did finding answers for these questions even matter now? The milk was already spilt. Why listen so closely to the echoes from my past?

What about the numbers of peanut allergy cases on the rise in certain countries around the world now? Thirty years ago peanut allergy was almost unheard of. Yet in 1995, Australia reported one in two hundred cases affected by severe allergy. Just over a decade later, in 2007, The Australian Society of Clinical Immunology and Allergy reported that the numbers of peanut allergy cases had doubled in size over the previous five years, reaching a staggering one in twenty children, and one in a hundred adults affected in Australia alone. This sharp rise wasn't only confined to Australia.

Recent medical research in Canada reveals one in thirteen Canadians suffer from life-threatening allergies. An epidemiologic study published in January 2011 in the *Archives of Internal Medicine* estimated that as many as forty million Americans may be at risk for severe allergies or Anaphylaxis. According to the Anaphylaxis Campaign in the United Kingdom, one in fifty children in 2002 were believed to suffer severe allergic reactions to peanuts, tree nuts, or both. That's one child in every second classroom. In 2002, the UK population of children under sixteen reached thirteen million. That adds up to a lot of allergic children and a far cry from the 50,000 allergic children reported only a decade before. At the same time in Ireland, statistics indicated that approximately 5% of children and 3% of the adult population had food allergies.

In February 2011, BBC News reported new research had found that boys were more likely to be diagnosed with a peanut allergy than girls. The study, published in the *Journal of Allergy and Clinical Immunology* by Edinburgh University researchers analyzed 2005 data from over four hundred English GP practices—nearly three million UK patients.

The report concluded that:
> Boys were more likely to be diagnosed with peanut allergy than girls, children from higher income homes also appeared more likely to be diagnosed. Babies and younger boys were up to 30 per cent more likely to be diagnosed than girls of the same age. However, the gap in diagnoses between the sexes narrowed as the children grew up. By the age of fifteen, girls and boys were being diagnosed at almost the same rates, and by the age of twenty-four, the figures were reversed, with more women being diagnosed than men.

According to the researcher Colin Simpson, the reason for the difference was still not clear: "There could be a link to the sex hormones, but we don't know for sure. The fact that at puberty there is a change could point to a link, but we need to do more work," he said.

Patients in the highest income groups were almost twice as likely to be diagnosed as those from the lowest income homes. There were 0.7 diagnoses per one thousand patients in the highest socio-economic group, compared with a diagnosis rate of 0.4 per one thousand in the lowest.

This appears to confirm the common idea that peanut allergy affects those from the middle classes disproportionately. Clearly, statistics reveal that there is an allergy epidemic sweeping through the world and that young boys and higher income groups are at higher risk of a peanut allergy diagnosis. Age and hormones seem to play their roles.

Even though I hold the greatest respect for the hard work and commitment researchers and scientists put in to find answers, I see in these reports an emphasis on looking at the effects of a problem. What purpose does finding out this information serve? To give evidence, to fund further research, to keep me stuck, to feel part of something bigger, to give hope that something is being done, to have someone to blame, to offer a temporary Band Aid while waiting impatiently for experts to deliver what they didn't yet know?

What is right? Wrong? Or are the answers only accurate for one particular group or nation and not for others who deliver contrary results? What should I believe? Or trust? What benefit was it to me to hear that the numbers of peanut allergy cases were on the rise? How was I to take these new findings on board? Sometimes I felt like the purpose was for everyone to feel more despair that peanut allergy is out of control, knowing our experts can't seem to stop it.

Who was asking these questions anyway? Did they know what it was like to live and breathe pain and rejection every day, to have allergy as a constant never-ending spiral of thought? Did they know what it was like to face this beast first hand? To feel its firm grip as it takes hold and squeezes your soul? Could they imagine what it is like to try to survive every second, minute, hour, or day of unpredictability and uncertainty, to exist on a different dimension than the norm of society? How can anyone answer questions about what they don't truly understand or know?

I pondered, "How is all this data going to help my path of discovery now?" all the while thinking about the questions I would like to have answered. I picked up a pen with my non-dominant hand and began intuitive writing in the hope that I'd learn more.

This is what I wrote:

"What is in a question? The answer.
But where does the answer come from? The question.
Are you asking the right questions to get the answers that you seek?"

"Of course. That's it!" I said to myself, realizing that every question asked has its own distinct blueprint for the delivery of a particular type of answer. If I ask "why" then I will get a reason or an excuse; "where" will give me a location, place or destination, and "how" will give me a step by step process or some instructions to follow. So if I want a set of instructions it would be pointless to ask the question "why".

Among the wealth of information surrounding me, this came as a revelation. I pondered upon this "asking question strategy" unfolding right in front of my eyes, so crucial to know on my journey toward healing.

From my personal development courses, I had come to realize that when I asked myself a question, whatever was filled in afterwards was something my subconscious mind had gone to work on immediately. Right! So this would mean that the question itself must be the compass that pointed the innate intelligence's attention to a specific place in the brain or body. To where it sorted through the information, worked out the best type of response, and delivered the answer as a physical sensation, thought, feeling, or perhaps even a dream.

If the answers stemmed from the "effects" of a problem, the information might be useful in its own way, but it might only point further down a never-ending path, and hold only a tiny piece of a solution or none at all.

Therefore, if there was any hope of finding the cause behind my problem, I had better know how to ask the right questions.

Over the next few hours, I researched the art of asking questions and learning styles to formulate a blueprint to use. My inner wisdom had been true in saying that the answers I sought were in the questions I asked. The question "What if" reminded me of a time when I had been asked this in a personal development course in 2003.

"*What* would you do *if* you knew you couldn't fail?" was a question that stood out. I can still recall initially finding it difficult to answer this, to get past or even fathom what life might be like without being overshadowed by daily limitations. My life depended on always staying one step ahead of failure. I couldn't afford to make mistakes—to fail. I might as well have been asked, "*What* would you do *if* you knew you were allergy free?" I'd be unable to answer without having any prior first-hand experience with allergy freedom.

With certainty this question would stretch my imagination beyond my impossible dreams. There was no other way I could answer this without using imagination and fantasy.

I was asked to write about my perfect fantasy day, about the kind of day that I'd have if I had absolute freedom, unlimited means, and all the powers and skills I had ever dreamed of. The instruction I received was to be outrageous in my writing and to go for it. Whether this exercise was just to feed a pipe dream or not, it did help me to move beyond the drudge of the daily limitations that were imprisoning me. When I look back now, this was a good exercise to activate the subconscious mind, to enhance and develop creative thinking and to stretch the imagination. Had my inner wisdom simply been trying to tell me that for any chance of finding a solution, then I would have to stretch myself beyond my normal way of thinking—to introduce "how" and "what if" into my dialogue with my subconscious?

How did my body somehow steer off the normal path to react to harmless food as if it were poison? *What if* I looked for other factors outside of peanuts that might have led to this? *If* peanuts weren't the real cause, then *what* was? Asking in this manner might reveal something I might have overlooked. Everything was pointing back in time to explore early childhood; however, this time I would go back with fresh eyes to retrieve the information learned from the past so that a path that went beyond the problem could be constructed from the subconscious's knowledge and intelligence.

Retrieving disjointed, distorted or faded memories of the past was not easy. These memories came to my conscious episodically and unexpectedly. Their arrival didn't follow any chronological order. This made perfect sense, as I believed that the missing pieces of the puzzle that I sought were floating, wandering, lost in time or space just waiting for their particular trigger to be rediscovered—to be resolved.

15

Family Matters and Mirrors

"Most of what our body learns as children we pick up from mirroring others or from conditions in our surroundings."

Journal Extract: Michelle Flanagan

I felt blessed that my friend Fritz had pointed my interests towards personal development, when at first I had no idea how influential his friendship would be on my healing journey. With all this new knowledge under my belt, there was increased hope that I could now decipher and let go of distorted mirrors of my past. That, by taking the next leg of my journey to early learning and development, I had a better chance of recognizing previously overlooked factors in my early surroundings that may have led to, or contributed to, the manifestation of disease and disorder in my adult years. One lesson in particular stood out above the rest which, upon revisiting, would take me on a journey back in time, far beyond what I had anticipated.

I hope I get to my course on time in this traffic, I thought, looking at the cars in front moving at a snail's pace. Impatient drivers were blowing their horns as if to say "Get a move on!" and condensation was building on my windshield from the rain.

What about the drivers? I wondered. Where are they going? What's happening inside their cars? Are they talking with others, just listening to the vibes on the radio, or singing their favorite song? How are they feeling? Are they happy, sad, or just impatient to get home after a long day at the office? They were encased in their outer shells that told so much about them, lending them a label, color, a status symbol: the truck for the worker, a sports car for those who like to move in the fast lane, or the old rust bucket for those living by simple means or not doing too well in life.

I couldn't help but notice the reflective sign illuminating the bumper of a large yellow truck in front of me: "If you can't see my mirrors, I can't see you." Just glancing, this sign might be passed off as just another of the many messages and symbols that bombarded my senses everyday. However, this would become significant.

Under normal circumstances, these conditions would have brought on frustration, but today I didn't care about the congestion. Instead I was more curious about tonight's meeting topic on early childhood development. Always interested in this area, I made sure that I left home earlier than usual as I didn't want to be late. Deep down I felt a glimmer of hope that maybe this class could give me more of an understanding on how I had come to be.

Soon I was at the school, hanging up my damp coat with the others, heading straight to the classroom, making sure to get a front row seat in order to satisfy my curiosity. It wasn't long before the introductions were out of the way, and my teacher jumped straight into the lesson.

"Tonight we are going to talk about things from the past, early childhood experiences, and how our characters develop into adults." Just hearing these words made curiosity resonate through my bones.

"Learning about childhood can be very mysterious because most of us don't have much memory about the early years. Does anyone know why?" he asked, pausing for a moment as if waiting for someone to answer. Thirty-five sets of eyes stared back at him—our faces were blanks. The room was in silence, but my mind was a hive of activity, tracing back in time to sort through and find my earliest childhood memories. Snippets of lingering moments bubbled to the surface—but most surfaced between large gaps of nothingness. Why did I struggle to remember? Why could I only trace back so far?

After a slight pause the teacher continued, "We don't remember because when we are children we move about the world with a different way of experiencing ourselves. When you try to look back now, most of you are trying to imagine what it was like from a different perspective, as an adult. Children are feeling beings and do not recognize what is going on around them like you do now," he said, with all eyes fixed on him. You could hear a pin drop if you listened for it, but rather all attention hung on his every word.

"When a child experiences the world, they do so from a feelings and sensations perspective. That is why memory sometimes gets lost, buried in storage because grown ups are not in that feeling state to recall it," he said.

I began to repeat in my mind what he had just said. "So if I learn to listen and decipher the various sensations in my body...a flutter, a hot or cold feeling, a gurgle, tingle, stiffness, tension...then I might be able to reconnect with some of the old once forgotten memories?" I scribbled this down as a reminder in my notebook. I knew this had some importance. I just didn't know what.

"Let's take a step back for a minute..." he followed with a silent pause. My curiosity didn't want to take a step back.

"At the time we are born, our experience of the world is one of safety and warmth, cradled in the arms of unconditional love...Right?"

We all nodded in agreement. I couldn't help but quietly chuckle to myself at the safety and warmth oozing from the elevator shaft the day I came into this world.

"Your early years are a time of intense learning of so many things: crawling, learning to walk, making sense of words and language, recognizing people and places. You are a learning machine, gathering information at a speed that can only be described as truly amazing," he said with a smile painted from cheek to cheek.

"As a child you perceived the world in accordance to what was happening around and within your body, whereas as an adult most of you see the world by who you think you are now, filtered through your beliefs, thoughts, and attitudes that have taken a lifetime to form..."

Weird chattering noises began to sound from the back of the class.

"Oh! It's Jeremy up to his childish antics again," I snarled in the direction of the back of the class. It was as if Jeremy always waited for the opportune moment to interrupt, just when the topic being taught was at its most interesting. Why was there always one that ruined it for the rest of the group? I thought, shaking my head in disgust.

"Oh! Please we are not in preschool," my internal voice uttered in response to his inconsiderate carry-on. Were his adult displays of childish behavior simply a billboard advertising that he was too set in the ways of his past, a Peter Pan reluctant to evolve into an adult and never grow up? Or was he just more in tune with the conditions of his internal/external environment, more tuned in to his feelings and physical sensations? Did this define him and why being in touch with his feelings was so important—dominant even? And why did he hang onto yesterday like there was no tomorrow…a child in an adult's disguise who didn't want to grow up? Like a child, he always seemed to know the right moment to seek attention. When attention hadn't been shining on him for a while, he'd do something really silly or obnoxious to get it. Any attention was good. It didn't matter if it was positive or negative—it was attention. Was it even attention he sought, or rather to feel the energy from others, to touch and be touched? I reasoned.

"Shhhhh!" a low persistent hum began to infiltrate the room. Jeremy's attention-seeking displays of what he believed to be funny had become annoying to others too. I felt relieved when the teacher gave him two options—be quiet or leave. He chose to stay.

The room returned to the way it was before the interruption, but it was far from peaceful. My thoughts were now a hive of interference, actively sifting and sorting through my memory banks. The search was on for gold at the end of my rainbow—my earliest childhood memory.

"Maybe I'll try this later," I thought, for fear I'd miss something. My ears intercepted and turned up the volume a notch— anything to drown out distraction to hear what the teacher had to say.

"As children we learn from the world we live in, whereas as adults we live in the world we have created. If a child's environment is hostile or angry, they learn to fight or run away. In turn, the adult fighter or coward lives in a world constantly in battle or in limbo and instability. If a child lives surrounded by worry, they learn to fear. If a child lives with fear, they learn to be apprehensive, and so on."

I scribbled the word "FEAR!!!!" in block letters at the top of my page. Beside it I wrote a note, "Revisit this later". But I didn't. My excuse had a sense of irony to it—I was too afraid to.

"Don't be fooled into believing that you can hide your true feelings from a child. Their bodies have heightened sensory acuity, like an antenna picking up vibrations in the air. Feelings have a physical representation—a sensation or physiological shift felt in the body…"

A discussion between the parents in the group began—sharing some of the experiences they had encountered with their children.

I didn't have children of my own. This conversation bored me. My thoughts offered something to do. I wondered if the teacher had been talking about the unexplained ability I had as an adult to sense danger in my environment. Despite my five senses being out of range to detect a potential threat—I sensed it somehow.

Had my body retained this "expanded awareness" capability since childhood because it was crucial to have enhanced survival instinct in my allergy-threatened world? I felt my world. Like that of a newborn in an unknown, strange and threatening environment—when survival is imperative it doesn't need to know your views about world peace, poverty, animal rights—your beliefs and attitudes. At the moment of impact this serves no purpose. Animal welfare would be the last thing on my mind if a crocodile was about to eat me.

I felt my mind wandering like a nomad, a hunter-gatherer on a quest for information about the world I lived. Were these feelings and sensations, this felt sense, just part of my survival mechanisms? Was it a heightened sensory acuity imperative for survival in the times of early man but cast aside and clouded in this century? My gut began to rumble. It wasn't hunger for food in the literal sense but for more answers. My gut told me that this train of thoughts was heading down the right track.

"Okay, let's try a small exercise," my teacher said, interrupting this train of thought. "I want you to write down or remember the first thing that pops into your head. What is that? Is it an image, a sound, a thought, a memory? Is your mind blank or is it overflowing with information? Calm or bursting at the seams…Write down whatever has sprung to your mind. Okay. Now I want you to try something else…take a deep breath, and as you exhale let your thoughts go…they won't make sense to you now…that's it…deep breath…exhale…let them go…now without thought I want you to close your eyes and scan your body for any sensations or feelings…slowly scan, starting at the tips of your toes…to the top of your head…Is there an area that is particularly hot or cold…that draws your attention…where is it located…go there now…does it have something to tell you? …Listen…Explore…Does it tickle…are there pins and needles…or even numbness…do you feel pain?…What is that sensation?…The sensation that got your attention… is it strong or weak?….is it moving or still…fast or slow…does the sensation have a shape…a color…are there any thoughts?…A memory perhaps…or even a message…or is your mind blank?…Does it have a feeling?…an emotion…do you even know?…Continue to scan your body for a few minutes…let it guide you...Great! Only when you are ready...I want you to slowly open your eyes, take a moment to come back to the room and record your experience in your notebook. Did you notice any difference between when your attention focused on your thoughts or when you recognized sensations in your body?

"The latter was a felt sense. The world of children is not a mental experience but a physical one—a felt sense," the teacher said.

I tried to imagine what it would be like if my mental slate of beliefs, learned behaviors and attitudes built over a lifetime had been wiped clean. That all I could do was to feel and sense my world. To answer this, I knew, would require a little bit of imagination. Strangely, as I thought of this, one of Einstein's quotes fired off in my mind:

"Imagination is more important than knowledge.
Knowledge is limited. Imagination encircles the world."

I finally understood what Einstein meant by this. If it wasn't for the power of imagination, I wouldn't be able to piece together some of the missing puzzle pieces or memories lost in time. Imagination could give me a sense of what something I had never experienced before or knew might be like. I had accepted that I wouldn't have conscious memory associated with certain life events, but I now realized that my body has been there through the ages, recording every single moment of my life. Imagination could be the glue that could bind together forgotten moments in childhood. If used appropriately, it could help to put some of the missing pieces together that had been buried deep in my soul. As I didn't want to miss any of the lesson I quickly jotted this revelation down and turned my attention back to the class.

My ears perked up a few notches as soon as I heard: "The average child born into this world is perfectly healthy, with all its organs functioning correctly. Even though the body always believes that it is doing the right thing, in early development it is more susceptible to going off track." My interest to learn more about early learning in a physical sense took precedence over my childhood explorations. I really wanted to get to the bottom as to why my life seemed to have gone so terribly off track.

"Okay, class, before we go into more detail about this, I'd like you to take a short break," the teacher said, as if to tease my curiosity. "Tea, coffee, and biscuits are available in the kitchen...the one with the allergies...you know who you are...don't go near the biscuits...they contain nuts...Okay, we will resume in fifteen minutes to discuss how the mind and body learn in the early years. This topic will be of particular interest to those with physical challenges...Please come back on time all refreshed and with a clear mind," he concluded. I decided to stay in my seat and wait rather than mingle with the rest of the group.

Before I could say abracadabra, as if by magic, everyone was back, sitting on their seats, refreshed and ready to pick up where we had left off. The teacher began to speak more words of wisdom.

"Before the break I told you that the body is more susceptible to going off track in the early years. This is why? What we learn as children, most of the time we pick up from mirroring our surroundings, and from cell memory passed down from our ancestors...Do you have a question Michelle?" the teacher said while reading my name tag, nodding his head in response to my raised hand.

"Did you say cell memory...meaning that cells remember?" I asked, intrigued. Out of all the material he had covered, I found this the most striking.

"Yes, I did. How do you think your immune system functions? If immune cells weren't able to remember viruses, parasites or any other threat for that matter, how would your body protect itself from the multitude of diseases, harmful parasites and bacteria, toxins and viruses out there?..." he replied. "The cells remember."

"So what you are saying is that our memory isn't just stored in our head, that we store it everywhere else in our bodies," I responded.

He nodded and said that this topic was covered in the lesson later and that I would find answers then. He then continued the lesson where he left off before my interruption, "As a child's body is in a heightened feeling state in its infancy, this means that the information it takes in or mirrors can easily get misunderstood, misinterpreted, interrupted, or altered. Their immune systems, designed to protect them, is still in its infancy; the mind designed to process information about the outside world perceives it through a felt sense in childhood, and children rely on grown ups for their survival, learning, and growth. They are like aliens from outside of their world, in a different time, space, and perspective. By the time we reach adulthood, our memories of a past event can influence and shape the way we think, what we believe, how we feel, our values, and how our physical body functions, even on a cellular level," my teacher paused for a few moments to give us time to process.

I found it interesting to learn that past experiences or memories are gradually forgotten, becoming nothing more than a hologram of broken mirrors that has built over time to create illusions of reality. I also learned that our body plays such an important role in the early years, that over time certain factors or circumstances can either strengthen or weaken specific body parts or functions, influence energy and blood flow, damage cells, and even lead to the manifestation of diseases or specific health disorders later.

I pondered: Maybe my body going off track could even be generational, that by simply "mirroring" along the way, a mistake was learned and passed on. By becoming more aware of who I was as a human being, I might realize what the misinformation was. Maybe part of being an adult is to learn to be a child again—to go "back to basics" to when I was a child, except this time with the extra wisdom learned in my adult years.

The teacher began to talk about how family can influence our development—that the influence can be generational: that certain characteristics or family traits can be subconsciously passed down through generations. These characteristics or family systems can not only affect family, but also our health, relationships, careers, groups, communities, organizations, governments, and even countries.

This class would come to a close, but my notes and a handout with some examples of family systems and their influences remained. These would end up in a box somewhere, marked non-allergy related, to gather a few years of dust until I was ready to revisit my past, when my interest was sparked to learn more about information distortions passed down through generations.

This would lead my path of discovery into the world of epigenetics, a new field of science that studies how the environmental factors and lifestyle of one generation can affect the genetic activity, and influence health, disease, and lifespan of another.

Up until now, I had always been under the pretence that if I partied too hard, over indulged, killed a few memory cells on a night out, starved myself to prevent an allergic incident, or gained weight during the course of my life, that whatever choices I made for me, that these could never change my genes—my DNA. That all the genetic information residing within, regardless of life choices would be preserved and passed down to the next generation. I was surprised and intrigued to learn that studies in this field of science suggested that this wasn't the case.

Scientists of epigenetics discovered that environmental factors such as diet, prenatal nutrition, stress, exposure to environmental toxins, traumatic events, can make an imprint on genes, a memory that is passed from one generation to the next while leaving the DNA code intact. Research suggested that environmental conditions such as changes in diet, exposure to toxins like pesticides or chemicals, or extremely stressful events experienced during someone's life, actually influenced the genetic "markers" that tell genes to switch on or off, to turn up the volume or to go quieter. New switching information, along with the DNA, was then passed on to many generations, thus creating a trans-generational environmental effect.

This meant that the diet of my grandparents and/or any epic event encountered in their lifetime could have a direct biological effect on me. My grandparents had been through war and food rations, changes to food manufacturing processes, the introduction of the oral contraceptive pill, social reforms, and many more major changes. And their grandparents survived the Great Irish Famine. No wonder my switchboard was all askew.

Science could now explain why specific diseases tend to run in the same family, passed on from one generation to the next. Had the environmental conditions simply turned the switch associated with a particular disease on, imprinting the memory onto the cells and then passing it on? Then would this mean that if the environmental pressure or influencing factors were removed, the imprints would fade or dissolve, and the DNA code would revert to its original programming. This theory made logical sense even though I was not a genetic scientist. But how? And was there a reset button?

Did my body even know it went so terribly off track in the first place? Or was the information already distorted from another space and time? If so, how could I access the switchboard—to reset the memory—to retrain the body? Everything pointed to changing the environment, both internal and external if I wanted to find some resolution. I would have to trust my body to reset the right switches, knowing more so than ever how much it relied on me to listen to its messages, to believe, to stay committed and to act.

Instinctively, I was drawn to mirroring. It is the predominant method of learning by babies and infants when they sense their world by touch, when their communication skills are primal and under-developed. Instead of asking about the world in which they live, they mirror it—their environment is their teacher. This made me wonder. Does our body also learn from mirroring what's happening on the inside, or is mirroring only limited to our external surroundings? If yes, is it possible to change the internal environment so that our body can relearn, even on a cellular level? Is mirroring a way to reset the switch?

I didn't fully recognize mirroring until 2005, when I witnessed it with my own eyes. It was when I went home to Ireland for three weeks, ecstatic to reconnect with my family after two years. More importantly, I was over the moon because I'd meet two new family additions. Paula and Mark had each had a new daughter since my last visit—the latest members added to our clan. Mark invited me over to his home to spend some precious bonding time with his daughter, then age two, and his son, age six.

Mark's house was situated on the outskirts of Dublin, on a hill overlooking open fields, a parish, village, and ruins of castles. It was a picturesque place against the backdrop of the Mourne Mountains, with the Irish coastline seen in the distance. This familiar scene echoed memories of my childhood.

"Aunt Chelle...Look, it is Chelle," said two excited young voices as I turned into the driveway. My niece and nephew's little bodies radiated absolute joy upon making contact, excited as if Santa Claus was coming to stay.

Immediately, my nephew grasped my hand to lead me into the living room. There for all to see was his pride and joy, a large yellow truck complete with a top loader to fill with dirt. It had bright flashing lights and was covered with reflective stickers.

In the corner of the living room lay a bright-colored children's rug on the floor. This rug had a two-dimensional print: it was an aerial view of roads, roof tops, a river, a fire station, a bridge, police and gas stations, and all other elements of a make-believe town. My nephew would sit on this rug with his toy cars and trucks, passing the day playing village life, limited only by his imagination. It was as if somehow the rug took on a magic of its own.

For about an hour, I reveled in their world of fantasy and wonder. My nephew directed traffic, I constructed road blocks, and my two-year-old niece watched and learned with all eyes fixed on her brother's every move. How both ages interacted was fascinating to watch.

Everything my nephew did, my niece followed in his footsteps only seconds later. When he scratched his nose, she scratched her nose. When he played with his large yellow truck, she wanted to do the same, a mirror copy of his every move. I remembered the sign: "If you can't see my mirrors, I can't see you" as I was witness to "mirroring" in its purist form.

What if my niece hadn't seen or heard my nephew's behavior? I wondered. Would she have acted the same way? Probably not!

I was interested and intrigued because I could almost predict what my niece was going to do next simply by observing my nephew's actions.

Later I researched this behavioral phenomena and found that in the mid '90s a research team at the University of Parma, Italy, discovered "mirror" neurons in the brain—tiny neurological structures that fire both when observing action and taking action. The neuron mirrors the behaviour of the other. In fact, just by observing someone go through a painful experience, the observer may also feel pain. I'm no neuroscientist, but this looked promising, knowing that there was a built-in learning mechanism at my disposal within.

Was this how our internal bodies learned? I was excited by the possibility that if I changed my environment, just maybe mirror neurons would instinctively fire and reteach my body. It intrigued me to learn that we are programmed to imitate or mirror from the time we are born—that this innate ability which science has now coined the Mirror System is crucial for survival, especially for babies during the first few months of their lives. I would also find it interesting that mirror neuron activity fires in the parts of the brain that process information about touch; integrates sensory data; guides our thoughts, actions and feelings; sequences repetitive movements; and governs primitive motivations such as hunger. Was it just coincidence that these areas of the brain had a particular connection with the environment?

In fact, even as adults we naturally, but subconsciously, mirror each other. We do this so much so that words, gestures, expressions, postures, tone of voice and speed, even tiny minute changes in another person's body such as the breathing rate, blinking eyes at the same pace, and so on, tend to be in sync. An example of this can be seen while observing two friends or lovers in deep conversation. Their body language is in sync; their posture, tones of voice, and breathing rates appear to mirror each other. They are not mimicking; rather they are in a subconscious rhythm with each other.

I had seen friendly mirroring take place following a time when I had an anaphylactic reaction from accidentally drinking from a friend's beer glass only to find out later that she had eaten prawns hours before. Determined to avoid a similar incident, I began to drink bottled beer, only to find some of my friends following suit soon thereafter. Not happy with this outcome, I changed my beverage again to the most unusual mix that I could think of: white wine and soda water in a tall glass with no ice and a straw. To my surprise, it was only a matter of time before my friends changed their drinks again and copied my latest concoction. I couldn't believe how powerful mirroring was.

Does this mean that negative emotions such as anger, jealousy, fear, worry, etcetera, can be transferred from one person to another without us even knowing? Does mirroring include physical and mental states? Could this explain why most people I interacted with seemed to be stressed out just like me?

And what about genetics? Is there a connection? Surely if we can learn from mirroring, then this Mirror System could also play a role in imprinting? Imprinting genes? After all, this system is crucial for survival—survival of humans in an unknown or changing environment, especially when incoming information is distorted, not yet understood, changed or missing. Had I had another revelation? Connected some of the dots?

I knew that if I was to create a supportive environment for healing, external influences in my surroundings such as friends and family were important. Recognizing this innate mirror system, I thought that a little fun experiment might be appropriate.

Over the next three weeks, I hosted three dinner parties in my home. I bought and cooked the food, therefore minimizing any additional stress, and I sent out invitations listing a set of rules that my close friends had to follow. Even though they already knew about my allergies and therefore were mindful of the risks, they were told that there was an on-the-spot fine if the word allergy, or anything related to it, was mentioned during the evening.

I nominated a door person for each dinner party (each time hosting a different group of friends). The door person asked each guest a series of questions upon entry from a pre-written checklist. They were asked such things as what they had to eat earlier, did they bring any items with them, and if so, the label was to be checked for approval or disposal. That way I didn't have to become involved in the allergy management process.

The key was to host an evening in a safe environment, to converse about something totally different other than allergy, and to experiment with mirroring by changing the environment to see how it affected my guests. Throughout the evening, I changed the music, served carefully selected food known to evoke specific moods, adjusted the lighting at times, continually checked in with my breathing rate and state of calmness or fun, burned aromatic candles, brought certain colors into the conversation, and adjusted my posture to see if anyone followed.

As the night progressed, my friends' responses to all the changes confirmed that instinctively we mirror each other without even knowing it. But it also illustrated how powerful the conditions of our environment can positively or negatively influence internal physiology, mood, thought processes, memory, topics of conversation, and dictate the way we interact with other human beings. It influences our general state of well-being.

One VIP hour per week thereafter was spent researching mirroring, and other hours were spent on creating different environments designed to encourage healing and growth both inside and out.

Limited only by my imagination, I found conscious mirroring to be safe and fun. It also gave me more control over my environment, which I once had believed was out of my control.

What I found most interesting is that mirrors can work both ways.

16

The Lifeline Speaks

"Take a closer look at your blood and there you will find some answers."

Journal Extract: Michelle Flanagan

I can still remember the day the thyroid disease became apparent. How could I forget the constant barrage of blood tests necessary to monitor its activity? And even though the disease had gone into remission, the testing would continue. There seemed to have no end to this new routine, juggling my schedule every three weeks to stop off at the nearest pathology clinic on my way to work to give another drop of me for analysis. Then a few days later I'd visit my doctor for the results. All these appointments were exhausting, but what could I do? I had to do it. Thankfully, as my health improved, the frequency of testing tapered. But all the while as I wrestled my schedule, I felt deep within my heart inner wisdom was telling me something. It hadn't been the first time. Just now I had no choice but to listen.

I believe I was about six years old the first time "the messenger"— my blood—came to catch my attention. I estimate this based on my brother being about three. Like most new or unfamiliar oddities, if I was supposed to receive a sign back then, my young heart didn't recognize it. My sister, brother, and I were young, because our bodies were small enough to lie on the ledge in the back of the car next to the rear window. Often the three of us would squabble over whose turn was next, to sprawl full length, horizontally along the back window. There was only enough room for one. It wasn't required by law to wear seat belts then as it is now. Every trip was a battle.

"It's my turn," whined my brother.

"No, it's mine," I snarled back at him.

"No, you had it last time, it's mine," interrupted my sister.

"Mum, tell them it's my turn," quivered Mark's voice.

The back of the car was now getting heated as the squabbling intensified. We were pushing and shoving each other to climb to the prize.

"If you don't stop now, I'm going to stop the car," my mum yelled from the driver's seat. Her words unnoticed. We continued.

"I'm warning you. Stop fighting or I'll leave you on the side of the road." It might have been the response of any frustrated parent.

"It's my turn," continued to echo throughout the interior.

"That's it! I warned you but you didn't listen," she screamed in frustration, squeezing her foot down on the brake until we came to a complete stop. The squabbling also halted.

I can still recall the looks of shock on our faces.

Hurried out of the car, the three of us stood, and the tears began to flow. I saw red when the engine revved and the car began to move away. I could smell the fear, and full of regret for not listening. Abandoned! How could my mum leave me on the side of the road?

Red intensified. I could taste it on my lips.

Fright had turned on the nasal tap.

It was blood.

I don't know what happened next except that like magic my mum was there with a tissue and a deep embrace. We climbed back into the car in complete silence.

Nosebleeds would become a normal stress response growing up. When times got too difficult to handle, the blood would flow. But it would also carry an intense phobic response.

I feared my own blood.

I couldn't touch it!

Smell it!

See it!

Or even talk about it.

Or absolute terror would ensue.

I didn't develop a fear of abandonment, but it did enhance a fear of blood through association with this stressful event and a build up of others from the past. This fear would follow me until I reached puberty. The start of my menstrual cycle left me with no choice but to deal with it. It was either that, or for a few days every month for the best part of my life I'd be a phobic wreck. But what I did know is that by the time I reached adulthood, the nose bleeds had been replaced with rhinitis (swelling inside the nose) during stressful times. My nose felt constantly blocked; I was unable to breath, smell or taste properly.

As soon as I was diagnosed with the thyroid disease and knew that constant blood tests were required, I brought this childhood incident up with my mum. I never forgot the nose bleed. As is to be expected, my memory of this incident had faltered, but the physical symptoms had remained. She did leave us on the sidewalk but her car only moved a couple of inches. She had no intention to leave us, only to put a stop to the intense bickering and squabbling. My nosebleeds had manifested before this particular event ever even occurred. Could this explain why my brother and sister didn't have the same response? Their medical history was different, as too their stages of growth and development.

As soon as mum told me the truth about that day, the distorted memories dissolved. Surprisingly, I could breathe again. I had never even thought possible how much control and influence distorted memories could have over my physical health. With this revelation I was ready to face whatever was necessary to monitor the thyroid disease.

The rigorous blood testing had begun.

As weeks turned into months, I began to feel like a walking pin cushion full of holes. But gradually, thankfully, my senses became numb to the prick, the sting, the inconvenience and the added stress and pain. All I knew was that constant monitoring of this particular autoimmune disease was necessary. This was especially true when the thyroid gland, a butterfly-shaped gland located in the neck, was under attack. The butterfly was flapping and screaming—the volume had been turned up to a hyper frenzy as if a child on a sugar high.

Despite my once normal routine being in disarray, I began to ask more and more questions about what all these blood test results actually meant, and I was genuinely grateful that my doctor took the time to explain. She practiced the art of supportive communication, a far cry from some of the uncaring, unsupportive, nameless patient-doctor relationships I had encountered in the past. Her extra efforts made all the difference—she was a teacher in her own right. I understood why my whole body had been put under investigation. Understanding was the sugar-coated pill to sweeten the sting of feeling like a lab rat full of holes. But in truth, if this disease was shy and hadn't come forth when it did, I would still most definitely be struggling today. Or more so, I'd be pushing up daisies from six feet under like a fallen soldier who had lost the fight. The disease had come as my friend, not my foe. It was another messenger from the core—and I had to listen.

If my inner intelligence had been trying to send a message at this disease's debut, it came loud and clear: "Take a closer look at your blood". I only recognized this because I was forced to. How could I not heed this sign when my whole routine had to pivot around putting the life fluid of my being under the microscope?

I was tired of sitting in waiting rooms, stressing if I'd be late for work. Formulating just another excuse for my lateness had become exhausting. And it was a new job, a chance to find my feet since my relationship with Andrew had fallen by the wayside. I didn't want to mess this up. Surely disclosure of the new condition would distract my colleagues from their daily allergen vigilance. I was relatively new and most didn't know that Anaphylaxis existed until I showed up. Cloaking the truth from them was hard work, but I knew that the benefits of keeping it under wraps outweighed any consequences. Pretending worked pretty well. Well, that's what I believed at the time.

But I wondered if my fellow workers were blind or just too polite? They never once mentioned my "hyper" state, a common symptom associated with Graves Disease. But when I think about it, only those who knew me a while noticed. At work this state was normal—as was my reputation for being full of beans, working crazy hours into the night, being excitable and upbeat. No human could possibly endure this pace. But I did! And now with the disease in remission, I feared return to what I believed as normal might be perceived as slacking off by those who saw these changes as abnormal.

As usual I sat in the pathology clinic conscious of time—flicking through the pages of a magazine while my mind wandered as a distraction to kill the smell of sickness, or to extinguish the build-up of anxiety festering within. "Will there ever be an end to this?" I sighed, glancing at a clock for the hundredth time—growing even more fidgety in my seat as it neared the time when I should be on the road.

"How will I explain if I'm late this time?" asked my internal voice. "Please, please, pleeeasssse, let my name be next?" radiated its silent plea in the direction of the medical assistant on one of her intermittent visits to the room—a ray of hope that the wait was over.

"Mrs. Jansen," she called out, looking up from her clipboard to catch a glimpse of the next person to move.

"Darn," the inner voice said under my breath, and as if my envy motioned an elderly lady to wake from napping, Mrs. Jansen rose, with all eyes fixed on her tortoise pace. It had to be a deception of the eyes, like a spell to freeze time. I knew this spell all too well, yet the slowness of it was alien to me. I'd journey through life getting from A to B but memory of the steps in-between came full of holes—like a video fast forwarded to the main event, the steps in-between or surrounding it were ignored, bypassed, or classed as unimportant.

"If only I could stop time!" I wished, tasting the hastened flurry of anxiety consuming my saliva. Anxiety was palpitating my heart like a whip to a race horse—go faster or you will end up as food for dogs. Being late this time would be inconceivable—I'd be dead meat. My boss would surely bolt down the hatches and tighten the noose that was already around my neck. I couldn't afford to take any risks.

My attention caught an irritating tingle raising a persistent call. I needed to pee. Badly! But not now! I'd miss my call. I'll hang on and pretend this untimely call of nature is but a dream. The sensation will eventually subside. It has to. Jiggling my feet as a distraction brought some relief. I just didn't like waiting, doing nothing, killing time. My body obviously felt the same. How could it not feel anything different when stress hormones raged to quench the timeless boredom? It had to be alert, forever vigilant or it could slip into death's embrace.

"My name has to be next," I summated, taking a head count of those remaining: a young mum with her two young children, a girl and boy about five and seven years old, respectively; an old man, bald and wearing tinted glasses while resting slightly on his walking stick; a pregnant woman reading a book on baby names, predicting she had about two months left to pick one; and an Asian lady sitting rigid and upright. The wash of worry painted across her face gleamed in defiance. I felt fear for her.

I couldn't help but wonder why she was here.

Some read while others sent text messages; the only connection to the outside came via their mobile phones. "Please switch off your mobile phone," read the sign on the wall—its message ignored. The beeps of incoming messages were soon replaced by the eruption of a bickering session. The two children, like thieves in the night, robbed everyone from their inner worlds.

"Stupid," the boy said to his younger sister.

"Am not," she responded.

"Are," he retorted, grabbing a book out of her hand.

"Am not," she said in a whiney voice, signaling tears were about to fall. "No! You are stupid," she said, slapping his shoulder, clearly copying her brother's words from before.

"Ouch! That really hurt," he replied, taking a moment before he let it rip.

"Stupid...stupid...stupid..." his response now in rhyme to a tune he had heard. Their mother stirred, her expression tense like a tightly wound coil, shuffling in her seat as if trying to maintain her own sense of peace.

A feeling of déjà vu washed over me. I had been through this before. I didn't want to go into it now. I really needed to pee.

"The wait shouldn't be too long now!" I said, convincing myself to hang on, to not let go." Thoughts of early toilet training flashed in my mind—when I was anxious not to let go and feared that blood would gush down the back of my throat and suffocate me.

"Oh! Please...it's too early for this noise," I muttered under my breath, now seeing red. This kind of noise is annoying even if you are a morning person. Growing more irritated by the minute as the banter continued, I needed a distraction, anything to deter me from the physical sensation about to burst in my groin. I glanced around the room at the sterile décor, the magazine stand, the old man, and then the pregnant lady with her book of names. My memories came to my rescue as recollections of the many names I had been called over the years.

"Ana-the-fat-chick."

"Nutty Irish girl.",

"Nutcase.",

"Nutty Shell."

"Nutshell."

"Peanut."

The long list of names infested my head space; attention from the physical sense shifted. Instead, names that associated me with my allergies—labels—other irritations, interferences, niggling utterances that some found amusing all came to me. They took only a second to blurt out but a lifetime to endure. I had always been unwilling to retaliate or express my displeasure for fear I'd hurt the name-caller. I couldn't bear the guilt if I did.

"Ana-the-fat-chick" did help others to remember that I was an Anaphylactic…and it was a bit funny, even if it was at my expense. I'd wrestle within, trying to justify this constant reminder of my daily battle—a billboard announcing that I was flawed. When announced often enough, each and every billboard or label infused and solidified as part of my unique branding, which was my identity—the greatest flawed diamond that ever existed. Eventually, the words "Ana", "Fat", or "Chick" heard on their own was enough to trigger thoughts and memories surrounding my plight; guilt over self-expression prevailed. Just the thought of saying, "No more" squeezed my heart and soul, stopped blood flow and slapped guilt into waking.

"Don't be *mean* to your sister," the mum finally addressed the squabble. "Sit here and stop being such a *baby*." She moved down a seat to create a gap for the sniffling pair.

"You are old enough to know better," she ranted at her boy. "I expect to see this type of behavior from your baby sister…but not from you," she snarled, abruptly grabbing her magazine to resume reading. Shamed into silence, the seven-year-old slouched on his chair, perplexed and still. His sunken eyes spoke of sadness.

His sister grinned at him in triumph. She won. Mummy had favored her. She wasn't stupid after all were probably the words going through her head.

I wondered if the woman was even aware that she too had entered into their bickering—that she was a name-caller just like them. Is this trait unknowingly learned in childhood and we are unaware that we carry it through a lifetime? That it stirs a bittersweet cocktail in us, making it okay to joke about or emphasize someone's shortcomings? Do we engage in this verbal abuse because it is programmed into us on a subconscious level as children and we don't recognize it consciously as adults? Is sarcasm or bullying just more of the same—except with a different mask? I pondered.

Jokes about serious diseases like cancer are taboo and insensitive, yet a life-threatening allergy seemed to be a laughing matter. The list of remodeled names came in faster than the spread of a thick fog through the Scottish moors. I didn't understand. My condition was serious, a killer in a world of disorder and rejection. Yet there was something funny about it to others.

Was there an unwritten rule in name-calling—one that told what human suffering was acceptable to make fun of? Was there some rule that gave the seal of approval to mocking that which is hard to understand? Or did this rule simply follow the distorted mirrors of the past—like an innocent puppet dangling on a string? Acceptable verbal abuse learned in childhood could be disguised as harmless fun in adulthood. Had I just become numb to its subtle twists and turns, the occasional jab, pain muted by time just like these blood tests—getting used to it gradually—failing to recognize the sting? And I took it. My pride overpowered feeling shame. The irony makes me laugh. Was laughing sending the wrong signal, even though I used it as a sugar-coated pill to mask the pain, to fend off the guilt of expressing the pain—did it unwittingly approve the abuse? I genuinely didn't feel any pain. This confused me.

The clock was ticking. I was bored and fidgety. The urge for the bathroom had subsided. I glanced around the room in search of a nice picture I could escape into. Instead of serenity I found shame—a "no smoking" sign on the back of the door caught my eye—now common signage in a public place. To my surprise, it triggered memories of Santa and Christmas, even though it was now June.

I drifted to a time when a company I had once worked for had decided that year to have a "Secret Santa". We were each to give one small gift to another colleague; as a secret Santa, your name was kept anonymous. With the festive season almost on top of us at the time, about thirty colleagues gathered around the Christmas tree, our secret parcels glistening under its dazzle and shine. Each of us chatted and drank to festive merriment while waiting for our name to be called. That was our signal to take center stage, to open our secret parcel in front of the onlookers.

"This one is for Michelle." I can still recall a colleague's words, as I was passed a brightly wrapped gift the shape and size of a tissue box.

"I wonder what this might be?" I said with a smile, rattling its contents to create a bit of mystery, intrigue, and a few smiles. It did, at least for a little while.

The unraveling began. First ripping the outer paper shell—all eyes fixed on what my Secret Santa had bestowed on me.

Then I halted.

I took a breath.

"Oh! I don't know what to say!" I uttered at first sight of the outer box. Some laughed. Others stood, perplexed or in disbelief. My Secret Santa had made an effort. But the first impression squashed any desire to reveal any more of the present. Blood flowed to my cheeks as embarrassment set in.

"How do I take this?" questioned the voice inside my head, puzzled what to do next. "Do I trigger a laugh to guard my heart from the pain and embarrassment this causes me?" An awkward smile began to form as my precautious defense went into gear. I wanted to leave the room but all eyes were fixed on the contents of the package.

The box's exterior read in bright red letters: "Peanut Allergy Survival Kit". It had a large red medical cross on it and there were red "No peanuts" symbols scattered all over it. It looked as if the box had caught the measles, and I felt repelled by it.

I cautiously removed the lid, revealing the box's inner secrets—a pair of latex gloves (luckily I wasn't allergic to latex), numerous band aids, a couple of face masks, alcohol wipes, and various other medical paraphernalia. I knew this was meant as a joke, but this had crossed the line, even if it was not meant to. Each item was a reminder of my daily struggle and held a toxic undertone. I felt it etch an even deeper crater inside my soul. I had become immune to jokes about my malady, but this day's joke was different. This gift had an aftertaste; it held remnants of an emergency still fresh in all of our minds, for it was on this spot a few months before that I had danced another traumatic dance with death. I bowed my head.

Early that morning, the unsuspecting killer had waited out of sight for its target, contaminating all things in the office by its deadly touch. It was just killing time before it showed its ugly face, but by then it was too late. My body had already been ambushed. The peanut had struck again, and the attack was in full view. For the first time in this job, it had raised its terrifying head to the same audience gathered around today. An allergic incident ensued.

Thankfully, my boss had set out to investigate, and by the time I returned to work a week later, a "peanut ban" had been implemented. The message was clear: "Leave your peanuts at home."

But what I was told would be even more disturbing, as it indicated a new turn in my illness.

"How are you feeling?" asked my boss upon my return.

It had been a very trying week—no surprise about that.

"Oh! I've been better," I replied.

As with every other emergency I had encountered, there was the aftermath, a fallout effect, a sticky residue that wouldn't budge. Death had touched my soul and left a psychological numbness that can only be described as being on an intense rollercoaster ride. The highs almost reached the heavens: I had survived—I was alive to see another day. But the dips were dark and bottomless and verged on hell—death had come too close for comfort and left an imprint. Yet I was sent home from ER, following four hours of observation after being admitted; I was left to deal with the huge mental and emotional ramifications of a near-death encounter on my own. How could the medical profession leave me to deal with something so huge? How could I be feeling all right, when I was still dazed and confused and in want of support and guidance? Did they even realize the impact a life-threatening allergic reaction bestowed? Once the lid is opened, it too contains an unsuspecting residue, not only for me but for onlookers.

"I've replayed last week over and over again in my head, trying to figure out how it happened," my boss told me. "But I couldn't think of anything."

My guilt stayed hidden. I had left my colleagues for a week to pick up my broken pieces. Who wouldn't feel guilty? I had let them down again.

"You've obviously noticed the 'peanut ban'," he replied. "You scared us last week, and we are happy that you are okay now. Two of our employees have a serious peanut allergy, so we've told everyone not to bring nuts to the office," he continued. "A lot happened after you left last week."

"Yes," I said. "I heard that you had everyone clean the office from top to bottom. I really appreciate it. Thank you," I replied, truly grateful for the efforts. I was a close colleague and friend to many. I knew they wanted to do all that they could to keep me safe.

"That's not all. While we were cleaning I brought in the office cleaners to help us. They were shocked and surprised to hear what happened. And…"

What I was to hear next would knock me for six.

"While we were talking, the cleaner mentioned a mess they had to clean up from the nightshift early that morning. The mess was peanut butter."

"What? Peanut butter. Where?"

"It was on a desk away from yours, but that was before they cleaned yours," he explained.

I didn't quite get what he was trying to say.

Then everything made perfect sense.

"The same cloth was used to wipe your desk."

I recall feeling happy to now have an explanation but afraid to take a breath, realizing how sensitive I had become.

The realization came like another nail in my coffin.

The daily battle had just stepped up a few notches. The suffocating box was closing in. Life's nails were tightening their hold. My allergy was getting stronger—going deeper under the surface, going incognito.

Despite the implementation of the ban it would prove to have one fundamental flaw. It came without any training or crucial knowledge about the condition that only a person living with it could know. Knowing what the constantly changing hidden codes on food labels meant, the mandatory vigilance that came with a death sentence.

"Michelle, can you check this label for me, please?" was a common question asked before lunchtime.

"What happens when you have a reaction?" was asked by another.

"Can you pick out the venue for the Christmas party and the office event?"

I was slowly becoming involved in the planning of office social activities because of my special situation. The questions kept coming, and I was grateful that everyone showed such an interest. I told them everything I could. I knew that education was the key to my safety. Perseverance reigned over exhaustion

This ban (or any other in the future) would feed a false sense of security. Mistakes were more prone to occur when no one really knew what to look for. The ban in an untrained, uninformed, and unprepared environment was like arming a ticking bomb that could go off at any moment. The risk of a medical reoccurrence actually had increased. So I spent a great deal of time indirectly training everyone on how to create a safer environment, ban or no ban.

I now understood why my Secret Santa automatically thought to give a "Peanut Allergy Survivor Kit". My peanut allergy had become the talk of the office. It was the main thing that people associated me with—it was my label and the topic of most of my conversations. My friends meant well by making light of my situation, but this made me feel even more alone, helpless even. My battle was with my allergy. There was no room for anything or anyone else.

"Miss Flanagan," the voice of the receptionist in the pathology clinic brought my attention back to the room. At last it was my turn.

As I made my way to the consulting room, memories of the first time I saw my blood from a different perspective flooded back to me. It was in 2003 when dad had urged me to visit his doctor for a consult during one of my trips back home.

"Doctor O. specializes in severe immune-compromised cases but what makes her different is that she practises in both traditional and natural alternative medicine," Dad said, his voice ringing with a glimmer of hope. Maybe her knowledge in both Eastern and Western medicine might shed some light.

Yet spending my time in a doctor's consulting room was the last thing I wanted to do on my holidays. But how could I say no when my heart strings were being pulled? Despite wanting to take a temporary reprieve from anything medical, the internal battle to satisfy the wishes of someone so close to my heart overruled—I gave in. I wasn't going to feel any guilt this time. But despite agreeing just to make Dad happy, I secretly decided beforehand that any advice from her would be ignored. Taking time to visit her was nothing more than an illusion. Was a "Yes" without intent a disguise for "No"? But saying "Yes" to something I didn't want to do was the sacrifice I was prepared to make rather than feel guilty for saying "No".

"I am only here for a short visit and any follow-on care wouldn't be available when I get back to Australia," I reasoned as my excuse not to do anything beyond the consult.

But that soon changed.

I can still remember the moment of amazement when Dr. O. pricked my finger and put my blood sample under the microscope.

"Wow," I said at the sight of my blood enlarged on a big screen. I had seen many pictures of blood cells in science books, but I had never seen a "live blood analysis" especially when the cells under the radar were mine. It was only natural that curiosity would get the better of me. Any pre-cursors set to ignore advice instantly dissolved.

"What are those circular discs?" I asked, pointing at the screen.

"They are your red blood cells." Dr. O. replied. "They pick up oxygen from your lungs and transport it around the body to every cell." I listened intently.

"Do you know your blood group?" she asked, filling in my medical details in the new file created.

The blank look on my face told of my answer.

"Your blood group tells you what type of blood you have," she replied, explaining how blood is classified into four groups O, A, B and AB and that it can be positive or negative, depending on the presence of D antigen, and how your particular type is determined by your parents.

"Hold on a minute, and I will ask your dad," she said as she left the consulting room to speak with him. Moments later she returned with a gaze that reminded me of Sherlock Holmes—inquisitive and on a mission to uncover some clues.

"Your dad tells me that your mum has a negative blood type and that you inherited the positive blood type from him…he also told me that you were born in an elevator," she said with a smile.

"Oh! He often tells everyone that story," I said laughing, totally unaware that what she had just said may have some significance. Instead, anxiousness to get back to the main topic got the better of me.

"I see from the form filled out earlier that you've had a lot going on over the years," she said, as she began to read out my long list of symptoms. This was my cue to switch off.

"Yes, but?" I retorted feeling overwhelmed and even more flawed hearing my history of ailments in one hit.

"This isn't what I want to hear on my holidays," I thought. Matters of my health, except for allergen vigilance, could take a hike on my holidays as far as I was concerned. I changed the conversation.

"What are those odd irregular shaped cells?"

"They are white blood cells—cells of your immune system that defend your body from disease and foreign substances," Dr. O. explained.

Over the next thirty minutes we talked about the immune system, metabolic types, nutrition and deficiencies, digestive parasites, vaccinations, free radical damage, and blood cells. I left with some guidelines to make some adjustments to my existing diet and knowledge that my blood showed some vitamin deficiencies, especially in the vitamin B group and that I was a bit dehydrated. I passed this off as nothing more that the effects of jetlag and increased alcohol consumption while visiting my friends. Even though I would revisit this later, the most unusual recommendation would stick in my mind: use of a small electronic capsule, a Russian medical device used to restore digestive function and metabolism, to zap parasites taking up residency in my gut.

"Waiting for my name to be called has proved productive," I thought, looking at my journal and recollecting some of my memories.

My list of new things to do read something like this:

Find out more about this name-calling trait. I would never have been called "Ana-the-fat-chick" if I wasn't an Anaphylactic to begin with.
How do I change this trait?
Tell my friends how I really feel when they call me names.
It is okay to say "no". The next time they call me these unwanted names, respond with a positive name or action that I want them to call me or to do...they will eventually follow/mirror.
How did my ailments get their names? Is there something more to learn from understanding more about medical naming conventions?
What else can I learn about blood?
Listen to my heart. It is trying to tell me something.
How can I use blood regeneration to my advantage?
Replenish kidneys—drink lots of water.
Cleanse the gut to repair and restore digestive function.
Contact Dr. O. to order another capsule.

After my blood was taken, I grabbed my coat and journal and made my way out of the pathology clinic.

"See you later," I said, knowing that I'd be back soon. As anticipated I had gone past my time. I would arrive late to work that morning. This time, instead of making up excuses, I would tell my boss the truth about the blood tests. For the first time I had realized that I had been doing more harm than good by trying to keep them a secret. My boss understood. In fact, she encouraged my wellness, adding some flexibility to my schedule.

When I look back now, the diagnosis of the thyroid disease had definitely come as a blessing as it had literally put my whole body under close scrutiny. This would become the fuel that powered my journey of healing towards the glands—the body's unsung heroes. I would also learn that one drop of blood held my entire history—the place where my allergy resided. I learned that blood type compatibility between parents can influence the baby's blood. Now knowing my parents' blood types, I could pursue a path to explore blood incompatibilty issues present at birth that may have gone unnoticed.

I knew that I couldn't change my blood type, but I could learn how it influenced my health. Regular blood analysis told me the truth, the here and now about my immediate state of health—the environmental conditions. As for the negative labels, I knew this trait could be changed, retaught, eradicated. That day I stood in front of the mirror and told myself, "No more". I made a promise to myself to stop hiding from the truth. It was time to stop avoiding what my heart had been trying to tell me all along.

To forgive is to let go of the past.
A forgiven past can generate compassion for others.
It was time to clear the pathway to the heart—to love.

17

Avoidance Can Be Futile

"Avoidance has two sides. On one it can keep you alive, but on the other, if left unchecked, it can subtly take a hold of your life, spread distress and heartache onto others, and can even lead to an untimely death."

Journal Extract: Michelle Flanagan

"Stay away from peanuts and other known risks at all costs to prevent a life-threatening incident." I can still recall the only medical advice given—avoid, avoid, avoid—and it was crucial to prevent an allergic reaction or even death. Yet, conditioned to avoid from a young age, over time I had learned that avoidance after trauma or stressful events has a deeper, more destructive side to it. Even though the act of avoiding was sustaining my life, it also had the power to sap it away.

Imagine if going to a restaurant or having dinner at friend's or relative's was a life-threatening endeavor. Imagine that simple everyday tasks such as brushing your teeth, having breakfast, feeding your pet, shaking hands with someone, or even greeting a loved one with a kiss might be death for you at any moment of any day.

It was for me.

By now I had a long shopping list of allergens to avoid. The only time I felt comfortable saying "no" without feeling guilty came with allergy prevention. The potent, useless, stagnant energy of guilt was automatically pushed aside to allow survival to step forward. Yet even though avoidance prevented an allergic reaction, in truth this advice from my doctors had become extremely difficult to follow. Core human needs (like eating) that kept me alive could also kill me. Gradually, over time, I had become so sensitive that even microscopic traces of the allergen were more than enough to set off a whole array of allergic symptoms. I put this down to the frequency of incidents.

I can still recall the time in my life when allergy prevention was manageable. Now I was just too sensitive. Death was getting closer. The risks were everywhere. Some were invisible to the naked eye, and they infiltrated human's most basic needs for survival—food, air, water, shelter and reproduction. Because it was a do or die situation, learning to avoid was a must.

But that wasn't all. As I ventured out into the world on my own, fear of having a reaction without anyone with me grew into a great need to make friends, to establish a footing away from home, to belong to a group for reassurance, security, and peace of mind. I was prepared to take the risk of rejection if it meant that I got this network of potential support.

As my sensitivity levels grew, so too did anxiety when I went out. It was a Catch-22 situation—I had become dependent on others to keep me safe, but going out to meet them put me at risk. Alcohol would become my vice to take the edge off social interaction. Rejection and social exclusion were everyday occurrences—the nature of the beast. And pleasing others and seeking acceptance haphazardly steered my path. I literally needed to belong, to be accepted, to be included. Belonging to something or someone defined me. It took the sting off the daily struggle. But the nature of the beast also had an internal physical mechanism, a learned behavior I didn't know about, passed on from our ancestors through evolution that served in a more destructive and sinister capacity in these times.

When I told most people that I was allergic, the preconceived idea was that I just got a rash, developed a cough, sneezed, or something simple, like a common cold. The reality was that if I came into contact with the offending allergens, I could have an anaphylactic reaction and possibly die. This scared most people, which often triggered an impulse in some to avoid me—to reject me, to leave me out, to exclude me, or to retract from me for fear of dealing with it. It was a classic example of fearing what we do not understand. With little known about the condition, avoiding it when it reared its head made perfect sense.

In 2001, even though I didn't know it at the time, I would witness another side to avoidance: the most destructive and extreme side of it:—a side that took my best friend's life.

John was my dearest and most treasured childhood friend. It greatly saddens me that it would take his death for me to recognize that avoiding allergens wasn't where I needed to look to find solace. I needed to look at the more destructive, deeper level of avoidance. I needed to learn to identify and rewrite the more destructive coping and survival strategies that had been imprinted in my life's guide book within. As long as that destructiveness existed, I had little or no chance of a full recovery.

"Michelle, John is dead," came the distraught voice of a dear friend, Helen, who called me in an act of bravery on a Sunday night in August 2001 to break this tragic news. I had met Helen in Munich. She later relocated to Ireland and, through my referral, became John's flatmate. We had become really close, trusting friends. Having my two closest friends under the same roof made me happy. I couldn't believe what she had just told me.

"You are joking, right?" I said, thinking that this was one hell of a sick joke to put anyone through.

My last trip to Ireland had been in 1999 during my case against the airlines; however, I had been in constant contact with John on the phone since. I can still recall the day during my 1999 visit when I pulled him aside to talk to him about his heavy drinking. Later, on my return to Australia, I was happy to hear that he had gone into rehab, was finally "on the wagon", and was getting his life back on track.

I can still recall our last phone conversation. To this day, I still wish I had listened more, knowing that this was his final goodbye.

One night in June, only a month before his death, the phone abruptly woke me in the early hours of the morning. I had been out on the town and a vicious hangover had already started to set in. Instead of ignoring the annoying sound, I knew that a call at this hour could be a family emergency, so I answered it. It was my dear friend John.

During the brief moments he spoke, he told me how much he loved me; he spoke of the special friendship we had, and said through slurred words that he missed me and wanted me to move back home. Angered to hear the drunkenness in his voice, irritated to have been woken for a senseless chat, my response was the last thing I'd say to him while he was alive. My words would bother me for years to come.

"Don't ever speak to me again unless you are sober," was my reply as I hung up the phone.

How regrettable and ironic these words proved to be. We never spoke to each other again while he was alive.

Alcohol had won.

It would take another three years to realize that I too was heading down the same slippery slope. I had become obsessed with being the last person to leave the pub. Moderation didn't even enter my mind during nightly binges of excessive imbibing.

I never learned to drive a car until I was about twenty-nine, but I never drove even after I knew how so that I could drink to my heart's content well into the night. I wasn't in conscious control; my subconscious was. Going into total oblivion was the preferred coping mechanism to push down and forget the pain of my life. I was afraid to feel difficult emotions. If I started to cry, I feared that the tears would flow forever; that if I unleashed the anger inside, I might lose control; and if I said "no", the guilt of upsetting someone else would spiral into more guilt. So I would party hard, laugh it off, sleep through it and wake up to a hangover, numbing the fact that another challenging day lay ahead. Alcohol had become the perfect method to temporarily forget about it all, to drift away, to stop time, to avoid facing my reality. Often I'd gauge how good a night was by how drunk I got. If I didn't remember the night before, it passed my gauge with flying colors.

Every time I had a traumatic anaphylactic incident, my alcoholic binges ratcheted up a level. Eventually, I was painting Sydney red more frequently; I was obsessed with going out and staying out whenever I could, to avoid being alone at home, to keep going no matter what, in order to cope. During the week, tea was my preferred beverage, but weekends always told a different story. I'd get wasted on alcohol.

Only a few months before the news of John, my mum had rushed to my aid when I was diagnosed with Multiple Sclerosis (MS). My life fell apart at that time. By the time she arrived, my coping mechanism had well and truly kicked in. I was drinking heavily to wash away the idea of MS. Upon returning home, she received news that MS had been another misdiagnosis on my list of many. But this experience did point out heightened activity and lesions in a certain part of my brain, the area associated with eating behavior. Could this simply have been a symptom of my allergies, only noticed when looking for something else? This would lead me to another avenue of unfoldment on my journey of healing when I revisited this part of my life later on.

My mother wrote me a letter, a helpless plea to stop drinking. Upon receipt I scrunched it up, buried it in my wardrobe to gather dust and ignored it. Alcohol had become a vice that kept the build-up of emotional turmoil and post trauma manageable. I wouldn't read this letter from my mother again until on my path of unfoldment.

Michelle, when I came to visit you I was shocked to see that you are drinking quite heavily. At first I thought that the drinking was a response to the MS scare but then one of your friends filled me with stories when I was there. This has added to my fear that something will happen to you and I am so far away.

I am terrified that you will get an attack and will be unable to recognize the symptoms because you are too drunk and end up dead somewhere. I am relying on your friends to keep you safe but I know that they can't be with you all the time.

I have gathered your friends' phone numbers so that I can contact somebody if I need to.

Please, I ask you to stop drinking so much.

I love you very much and worry even more about you everyday. Please get whatever help you need and call me anytime of the day or night if you want to talk.

Lots of love,
Mum xxx

I was in my mid-teens when I first tried alcohol, experimenting like any normal teenager. I was at an impressionable age, wanting more than anything to find my own place in the world, to fit in. I took risks like most teenagers to gain approval, but mine were toying with my life. My group of friends took turns stealing alcohol from our parents' liquor cabinets at home to drink before or smuggle into the teens' roller disco held locally every Saturday night. Yet alcohol wouldn't become my preferred method of coping until a little later.

I had art and fantasy as avenues of relief, regularly drifting off into my own fantasy world filled with bright color, paint, expression, imagination, and freedom. By the age of fourteen, drawing and painting horses had become my passion. I was even building my own little business enterprise selling oil paintings at a local hotel. My only desire was to go to Art College when I finished school, a life-long aspiration, a seed planted in early childhood.

I attended the largest girls-only convent high school in Ireland, situated next to the biggest cemetery, which is fondly called "The Dead Center of Dublin", and the National Botanical Gardens full of flowers and wonder, beaming with life.

Strong religious order, lots of prayer, strict rules and discipline were the teaching methods at school. Life was about duty, sacrifice, and to be of service to God. For a teenager already feeling imprisoned, without a mentor or anyone who understood me, this system proved detrimental to my development.

"I've given you history instead of art," the career guidance nun said when picking my class subjects.

"But I need to take art class as a prerequisite to get into art college," I replied, knowing that creativity was my only means of escape.

"Art is for stupid people." I can still remember her saying that and feeling distraught that her opinion could have so much influence on my life.

That day, any hope of making it into Art College was crushed.

I became increasingly trapped and stagnant, as if stuck in purgatory somewhere between the living and the dead. I was angry at God for so much suffering and pain. When I repeatedly failed Bible studies, the principal head nun singled me out as "Satan's child" in front of my classmates, isolating me even further by forbidding them to speak to me. Her name-calling had come with a vicious bite. I would hold the painful isolation from my mum for three weeks—then I broke.

"Michelle, is everything okay at school?" I can recall mum asking one evening after school. My silence told her something was wrong.

"Everybody is afraid to be seen with me," I replied in tears, yet relieved to finally tell her about the new branding—"Satan's child". As if a dam burst, nothing could stop the words flowing from my mouth as I spoke of the pain, "My friends meet me in the dark corridors...they are afraid to be seen with me...my desk has been singled out from everyone else—placed right at the front of the class...teachers pick on me...they think that I am a problem, a troublemaker..." I continued until I was blue in the face with exhaustion. The next day I was surprised to see Mum and the head nun enter the morning class. Mum had come to defend my name, to right the wrongdoing, to wipe the slate clean. I was singled out again, but this time it was to receive an official apology in front of everyone, telling all to call me by my birth name, Michelle, Hebrew meaning "Who is like God."

"Thanks, Mum," I remember thinking—wanting to shower her with hugs right there in front of everyone. She had vanquished the pain. News about the ban being lifted spread like wildfire through the school. Everything appeared to return to the way it had been before—except I was wounded.

In truth, the outward display of disinterest that teachers saw was the opposite of what was really going on within. I was struggling to learn lessons that seemed irrelevant or inapplicable to me.

I began to dodge school, to rebel against an institution that didn't support my needs. When under extreme stress, unbeknownst to Mum, I'd wave goodbye when she dropped me off at school, wait until her car was out of sight, then hide in the cemetery. There I would ponder the gardens, or aimlessly take a bus around Dublin for the day—anything to prevent adding more alienation or stress to my life. It would only be a matter of time before my cloak and dagger routine was found out. Only then did the necessity to move me to another school become apparent.

Located in the center of Dublin was my new co-ed school, the place where I met John. Often we'd hang out after school with a newly formed group of friends. Finally allowed to study art, the attainment of my aspiration to go to Art College was in sight. I was happy. John became a really close and trusted friend. It was as if we were joined at the hip, sharing some classes together, talking for hours on the phone, but he also held a darker secret.

In the early years of our friendship, I had two acute allergic reactions: one to a bee sting and the other to peanuts. At that time, the reaction time took about an hour and a half to fully materialize, and on both occasions John was there to hold my hand and get me the medical attention I so desperately needed. He saved my life both times. Someone saving your life is something you can never forget, especially to have saved it twice. Not wanting to add any extra stress or worry on my parents, as they were now separated, I withdrew further from anyone close to me so as to hide my secret.

John became my main confidant and trusted friend. Avoiding spending time at home, alcohol replaced art as my preferred method of escape. It was the most obvious choice to wash down my troubles, given that I came from a pub culture. Every time I encountered a traumatic medical incident or stressful event thereafter, I'd reach for the bottle and got drunk. My reaction to John's death was no different. But this time, the bottle touched on an intensity raging so deep within I was unaware even existed.

"Time will heal the pain," said a friend when we were out the following night. I was still in shock at John's passing.

"This is for John," I replied, raising my glass to celebrate the life he had lived, the times we had shared. I was confused when I felt anger begin to stir within. I didn't know how I was supposed to feel. My emotions were in conflict. I hadn't been present for the events surrounding his passing or there to hold his hand. I felt guilty to have done nothing to save his life when he had saved mine. The news of his passing came as disbelief, shock. I should have felt sorrow but instead I was angry, furious even. Angry that John had lost his fight. That I hadn't been there for him when he needed me the most and that my last words to him were spoken in anger. If he had been looking down on me that night as I raised my glass, he would have surely cringed to see me holding hands with his killer.

Over the years I had become afraid of angry, hostile or argumentative environments. There had been enough trauma and pain in my life—I just wanted peace. I hated confronting situations and therefore avoided them like the plague. It was easier to push anger down, suppress it, bury it as deep as I could—to avoid conflict at all cost. Conflict only brought more suffering and pain into my life. To grieve meant to confront anger, to confront anger led to hurting, to hurt meant to feel guilt. I couldn't do it.

Alcohol was my ally in freezing hell over for the next few years. How could the pain heal when my ally anesthetized it and helped me avoid it? I was afraid to let go of its grasp; if I did, hell would thaw. But by hanging on to it, I was only masking a stagnant, more destructive force in its wake. My life was conflict. My situation was delicate and fragile. By avoiding conflict, I hung onto the pain. I avoided living to my full potential. This gave the perfect excuse to party hard, take risks, hang on, trance out, and do whatever subconscious sabotage was necessary to kill the pain.

This would become apparent when out on a night out after diagnosis in 2004. The new developments in my health had forced me to take a break from alcohol for a while. On this particular night I was sober as I observed a friend of mine go through her own pain, helpless to do anything except keep her from harm's way. The despair I saw as it surrounded her body, unwanted feelings trying to bubble up to the surface of her being. It's easy to wash them down with the perfect numbing medicine, mirroring my own frantic effort to consume every drop of alcohol from the end of each glass, as if convincing myself that this was fun but knowing it was only a temporary painkiller. I could sympathize with her, but others watched her stumble and fall, slur her words, and they observed her as easy prey, those who look for their next victim.

To be a victim can be an interesting role to play. I knew this role all too well. Most of the time you unconsciously seek other people with problems, or you put yourself into compromising situations that you have little or no control over. Rejection comes as evidence to satisfy deep inner beliefs of feeling unworthy, useless, unloved, unappreciated, or defective in some way. I had to please. Rejection and "missing out" had become second nature to me. I was surprised to find scientific studies reveal rejection and social exclusion actually register physical pain in the brain and body on a subconscious level—that a lot of little unchecked events can turn into one great physical trauma. No wonder I numbed myself to any pain. No wonder I had to please others. No wonder becoming aware of this got me thinking.

"Do I follow the same destructive path to avoid my own pain, and why I don't feel it is because I have mastered avoidance so well?" I thought, recognizing this destructive pattern when my memory flashed back to the nature of my best friend's death. I came to realize that I was heading down a similar path.

Avoidance was my defense mechanism—avoiding allergens kept me alive. But I would learn that this is also a learned behavior that is passed down from our ancestors to ensure our survival. It was only natural for my clan or tribe to pass on this crucial survival strategy, taught from an early age to avoid threats or pain, to stay away from uncomfortable situations, or to fear what we as humans do not yet understand.

From childhood, my mind and body had been programmed to recognize and avoid potential threats or anything that might pose a danger to my existence. I learned about the risk or threat so that I could avoid it, and I'm not just talking about allergens. Like every other infant, I was told that such things as ingesting poison, drinking battery acid, or inhaling deadly toxic fumes can be fatal. I received warnings that swimming in crocodile-infested waters put me on their dinner menu, so it's wise to stay out of the water in such areas. I was conditioned to avoid the most obvious threats to my survival, but I was also guided, as a precaution, to avoid things I did not understand.

Avoidance is so engrained in our psyche it can emerge from the depths like a chameleon in different forms such as to reject, exclude, leave out, bully, single out, deny, forget, cast out, engage in hyper vigilance, self-sabotage, dissociate, ignore, to have selective hearing, to engage in substance abuse, experience sensory and time distortion, and trance out. These methods are all part of the same pattern—that is, to avoid. I thought of the mirroring system and wondered if this covert side of avoidance was simply a subconscious method to deflect pain from self or others—to avoid pain at all costs.

Echoes of this coping mechanism infiltrated every area of my life, manifesting in my behaviors, my thoughts, emotions, and social interactions. Formulated in my own inner guide book on how to deal with the risks and every day stresses of modern day living. I was sublimely taught through what I picked up from TV, the beliefs or advice of others, my culture, nature and nurture, and even through the language I spoke.

"Don't dwell on it", "Put it behind you", "Let's not go there again", "Stay away the next time", "Laugh it off", "Take a pill", "Let's get drunk and forget about it", "Turn your focus to your work", "Go shopping and pamper yourself", "Take a gamble", "Ignore it", "Break ties", "Run and hide": these are just some of the subliminal messages that we become so accustomed to. They have been built into our psyches somewhere along the way; imprinted into our own personal life guide books on how to cope with stressful situations, how to get through traumatic events, and, ultimately, how to survive.

When I realized this, I understood why my doctors' only advice was allergen avoidance. They don't yet understand acute allergy, but they do know the threat—the suspicious allergens that may trigger the condition. With no medical cure available, it's only natural that avoidance of triggers is the only recommended action to prevent manifestation of the allergic response. They advise patients to avoid, yet they rarely consider the impact this has on daily life—how it increases levels of anxiety and fear, thereby promoting favorable conditions for allergy to manifest, and how it increases risks in the environment.

I had a Catch-22 situation on my hands. It wasn't possible to simply stop avoiding allergens. That would put my life in jeopardy. Not avoiding would surely be an act of suicide, and therefore forever remaining vigilant was the only option. But I needed to make changes in my life to heal. Imperative as avoidance was to sustain my life, I had come to realize that when it's the main way to cope it interferes with emotional recovery and healing. How could I get past this challenge: to allow recovery and healing while still maintaining allergen vigilance? I found that gradually, over time, avoidance fed like a leech lurking in the shadows, insuring more pain and sucking my life dry. Maybe this was where I could turn my focus?

Avoidance and coping strategies had had a double whammy effect that was imprinted in my life's guide book within. Given the nature of this deadly beast and the intense fear and anxiety felt by all, everybody's focus, including mine, steered all teaching, advice, and actions towards what I couldn't have rather than what I could: "You can't eat this, can't go there, can't do that, can't, can't, can't, avoid, avoid, avoid."

Gradually, my subconscious had learned that anything that was uncomfortable, anything that I did not understand yet, even non life-threatening stressful situations, should be added to the list of things to avoid. This included conflict, feelings, getting too close, social interaction, commitment, and so on. Nobody had taught me anything different. Thus, most connections to what I believed I could have—joy, love, success, peace, freedom—were severed in my mind's eye. By the time I reached adulthood, I had become the Queen of Avoidance in EVERY area of life, and it was slowly killing me.

I would come to recognize that avoiding intense emotions may be the easier and most effective solution for short term temporary relief, yet over a long period of time, the emotional intensity gets stronger. It was as if my inner intelligence was "fighting back" to get attention, yelling at me to experience and listen to the emotion that I was avoiding. But I was too determined and stubborn, and I refused to stop avoidance. I had been taught this strategy from an early age as the only path to survival. Why would I wish to change this? I believe this is why I had turned, on a subconscious level, to a more drastic, unhealthy, and damaging approach like substance abuse. There was a sense of irony that self-sabotage had become the painkiller of choice to combat the pain of constantly having to avoid death.

Following many destructive avoidance strategies in my life, combined with constant rejection over the years, meant that an increasing build-up of unresolved trauma, unacknowledged pain, and anxiety lay festering under the surface, weakening my immune system. No wonder my immune system was in disarray. It would eventually explode as the manifestations of other diseases. What might have given rise to early cancer and thyroid disease somehow made perfect sense. These parts of the body had received the full force of the trauma on that terrifying night when I was raped over a decade before. Unchecked pain had already turned into trauma, and adding more that night only sealed my fate. As the trauma had never been fully resolved, I believe now that the trauma simply got trapped, shifted, or was buried on a deeper level. The cells distorted as reflections of the changes in their environment—a result of displaced energy trapped deep within the muscles, unable to move.

Could the non-life threatening avoidances in my life simply be efforts by my unconscious to prevent further injury to imbalances in bodily functions by changing conditions caused by unresolved, displaced, or suppressed energy—trapped pockets of intense e-motion, energy-in-motion—bashing against cell walls?

I would look at what I avoided with fresh eyes. As too what I believed I couldn't have or do. In simple terms I would come to realize that my avoidance patterns were simply markers to tell what parts of the body my subconscious was working on to protect me. This insight would take my journey to specific emotions and how avoiding these can injure certain bodily parts and their functionality.

For the first time in my life, I had lost someone close and dear to me, my best friend. Because alcohol had been his killer, I finally learned to grieve without the bottle. I remembered the many good times we had shared together. It allowed me to laugh, cry, love, forgive, let go, and heal.

Then I knew that if I wanted to find happiness, I needed to weed out the layers of non life-threatening avoidances, one by one, by changing my emotions, diet, thinking, and spirituality.

To uncover and release the destructive side of avoidance, I would have to look at the times I laughed things off or found a joke in the midst of drama because just under the laughter lay the pain. I needed to release years of bottling things up by allowing the tears to flow, to forgive myself for any regrets, to embrace what I could do rather than suffer because of what I couldn't, to not be too hard on myself for the many drunken nights of mayhem, for hurting my family.

I needed to start a new relationship, to fall in love again, except this time I needed to start a new relationship and fall in love with myself—to let go of attachments or expectations and just be. I needed to give myself permission to allow the pain to heal.

For the first time after many years, I picked up my paint brush and palette of color and began to fill my canvas with a new picture of life, thus replacing a destructive avoidance pattern with a more creative means of release.

John had saved my life on a number of allergic incidents, but he made the ultimate sacrifice of all: his leaving. When he left this world his passing taught me the most valuable lesson of all: to let go!

This is what saved me.

18
Love, Sex and the Power of Improvisation
"Let's talk about the stuff you don't normally tell your parents."
Journal Extract: Michelle Flanagan

It takes a confident person to get their wishes met in the clumsy exploration of having sex for the first time with a partner. I am one of those confident people (on the outside anyway, but there was always an interference buzzing through my head preventing total lack of inhibitions) that savors the art of making love and goes to extremes to make sure it continues to be a pleasurable experience.

By extremes, I mean all the daily routine questions: "What did you have for lunch? Did you brush your teeth? Anyone near you eat peanuts today? Can you change your clothes just in case? Did you wash your hands? What aftershave are you wearing?"

My partner was almost always someone I had known for many years; he knew me and he knew my allergy and he didn't want to be responsible for an anaphylactic incident. Our pleasure and my survival depended on these questions.

I can recall a Valentine's Day sometime in the late '80s early '90s as my boyfriend and I sat on a park bench showering each other with love, including additional intimate and awkward moments in a never-ending quest to live a normal life.

Cupid's celebration was spent holding hands and cuddling on the park bench, arms around each other occasionally brushing against sensitive areas of the body. The heat building between our bodies kept us warm on the brisk February day. And as my lover nibbled on my ear, a sigh would escape from my lips, with my eyes fluttering open and shut in lust.

Then I saw a smiling woman carrying a beautiful royal red box shaped in the form of a heart with a big silk bow adorning the cover. Chocolate! I really wanted my own Valentine heart filled with chocolate. But I had to avoid chocolate because it might contain peanuts. Whether it did or not, I had to avoid it just in case; you never know.

Early sunset prompted my boyfriend and me to move on from our leisure to get home and make dinner. But he had more than one surprise planned for me today.

"I want to make a detour on the way home," he said with a smile as we walked through the gates of the park.

"But I'm hungry. You know it's not safe for me to eat out," I replied, a bit frustrated as the familiar starving feeling from only eating at home had started to set in.

"It's already taken care of...you will just have to trust me."

Holding his hand as I pouted my lips in defiance of where he might be taking me, I kept my mouth shut as I didn't want to ruin what he had been planning for me on this particular day. Turning the corner, the famous arches were in site, an international fast food restaurant I had researched well and patronized whenever eating at home wasn't an option.

"Not here!" I said feeling a bit deflated because I wasn't getting any special red carpet treatment on this day of love. "I thought you were going to cook something special for me at home?" I said under my breath as we walked through the doorway into the familiar yellow and red plastic surroundings.

"Table for two?" said one of the staff, as if waiting behind the door to greet us, wearing a makeshift dickey bow, carrying a clipboard as if a host in a posh restaurant. I was confused. Am I in the right place? I wondered. My boyfriend looked at me, eager to see my response, especially the moment I saw a table in the far corner laden with a fine linen cloth, with a red rose, envelope, and a lit candle as the centerpiece. Even though the table was a bit out of place amidst the plastic and bright lights, that didn't matter as it was obvious he had taken some time to carefully plan this very special and comical dining experience.

"We'll have two burgers, medium fries, and cokes," my boyfriend said, placing his order with the makeshift waiter pretending to scribble on his clipboard.

"Oh, my God—this is so funny! How did you even think of this? It's brilliant," I said, laughing as we waited for our meals.

Given that it was a fast food establishment, the service was excellent, especially when our meals came complete with plates and cutlery, salt and pepper shakers, a bit of fun, thought, and lots of love. It was a first not to eat this kind of food with my hands. He had really made my day, but I would soon find out that there was more pampering in store later.

It wasn't long before our meals were finished, we had made our way home, and were cuddled together in bed.

The bedroom was lit with candles strategically placed on the dressing table across from the bed.

"Roll over, I have a surprise for you," my boyfriend said.

"What are you doing?" I asked.

"You'll see, roll over," he replied.

So I rolled onto my stomach and rested my chin on my crossed arms. My boyfriend got out of the bed and walked over to the candles. As he turned, I saw a brown bottle with an antique-looking label. As he approached me, twisting the black top off, I couldn't stop myself from asking, "What is that?"

With a sly grin and a quick eyebrow raise he slurred, "Massage oil. I have been warming it by the candles."

Lifting my head off my arms, I asked, "What kind?"

Flipping the bottle around, he read the heading on the label: "Aromatic Evening Primrose Oil."

"Does it have an ingredients label?" I asked reaching for the light on the nightstand.

"I asked the clerk if it was okay for allergies," he responded defensively.

"It's okay, baby, I just need to make sure it doesn't have peanut oil in it."

"It says Primrose oil."

"Yes, but is that the carrier oil, or the essential oil?"

"What's the difference?"

"Here, give it to me," I said a little too sternly, "Carrier oil is what they use to put the essential oils in. The fragrance comes from the essential oil. If it isn't mixed in the carrier oil, it can burn the skin. Some carrier oil is made from nuts. I have to check!"

He screwed the top back on as he handed me the bottle and I rolled over, tucking the sheet into my armpits in an attempt at modesty as the light switched on.

Holding the bottle under the bright light, I read the tiny print under the ingredients.

"The list is okay, nothing about nuts, but I'd feel better if you use my organic caster oil. I hear that it is good for the skin!"

Pleased that we could continue with our erotic foreplay, I turned the light off and snuggled back down on my belly.

My boyfriend opened the bottle and poured about a teaspoon full in his hand.

"This one is cold," he claimed in what could be called a whine.

"Just rub your hands together to warm it up, sweetheart."

Settling down and inhaling deep breaths to relax, I waited in anticipation for the oil to be spread on my back.

My boyfriend placed his hands over my shoulder blades and pressed down. The muscles on either side of my spine instantly responded to the pressure.

"Mmmmm, that feels good."

Slowly he began circling with the heels of his palm, gently spreading out over my shoulders and up my neck.

"That is so nice, sweetheart."

He pulled his hands back down my neck and onto the sides just under the arms, gently pressing his finger tips into the flesh beyond my rib cage and onto my breasts. Just a tease, though, just a slight tickle as he cupped my bosom. The massage continued as he moved up and down my back onto the top of my thighs. Again, teasing, but not touching the folds of my body.

"What a beautiful day, darling," I whispered.

My boyfriend slid his body on top of mine until he could nibble on my ear and whisper, "There is more to come, my love, turn over."

Reluctant to disrupt the sensual feelings created by his touch, I shuffled the sheet so it wasn't twisted under me. He had gotten off the bed and replaced the bottle of oil with a small jar.

"What do you have there?" I asked.

"Well, I didn't think you wanted oil on your face so I got moisturizer. I want to caress you from head to toe."

"Where did you get it?"

"What?" he said, as if he didn't believe I was asking such a question.

"Is it mine or yours?" An uncomfortable but familiar knot of anxiety was forming in my gut.

"Yours, the only kind you allow in the house!" he replied a bit sarcastically.

"I'm sorry, babe, but you know why I ask." I was the defensive one now. "I have to check it," I sighed, reaching for the light.

"Don't you trust me?"

"You know I do; I just don't want your efforts to go to waste if there is peanut oil used in it," I reasoned, "I have to be sure or I can't enjoy this!"

"You sure know how to make a man work to please you, my little Leprechaun!"

Flipping the light on, I stretched it under the glare to scan ingredients again. Quickly turning the light off, I handed him the jar and, with a sexy smile, said, "This is a first for me. I have never had a facial!"

"That's not all you are getting, my love!" he replied, determined to take charge of the situation.

My boyfriend proceeded to make me feel like I was floating on a cloud. How this man could turn me on by caressing my face was a mystery, but he did!

He started with my brow, pressing away the worry lines in my forehead, slowly moving to my temples, releasing the tension that had returned to my neck and on to my collar bone. I felt myself lifting my chest to meet his touch.

"Not yet, baby, I have something special for you there!"

Curious, I watched him move through the warm candle light over to the table, bringing yet another container of mystery substance to our bed.

Giddy with wonder, I propped up on one elbow as he opened the brown liquid and prepared to coat my breast for his feast.

"Chocolate? No, no, you can't!" I was crossing my arms in front of me as if fending off a deadly assault. "What are you doing!"

"There aren't any nuts in it. It's liquid; I got it at the sex shop," he protested, clearly not understanding my fear of his display of romance.

"Chocolate can be exposed to peanuts even if there is none in it. I have to do some research first before I can use this product. You know this! What were you thinking?"

"I was thinking I would please you eating it off your body. I'm sorry!"

"Okay, I know you meant well, but we can't risk it. Put it away now and please me without it!"

My boyfriend put his arms around me and apologized again.

"I do know better, I just wanted to give you a special day. I wasn't thinking with my head."

His caresses and kisses brought me back into the heightened state of arousal when he reached into the drawer of the night stand then reached above me to tear the package releasing a condom.

"Ah, babe, can you turn the light on?"

"Why now?" he responded with patience.

"Do you have the right condom?" I asked.

"I think so," he said.

"We need to check. Which one do you have?"

"All I know is the damn thing is Paddy Green!" he said, grabbing the sheet and walking out of the room, frustrated and in a huff.

"Come back. You know I have to check everything," I yelled through the door in an attempt to bring the pleasurable moment back. But it had been lost in the blink of an eye. Now I was on my own, on Valentine's Day, left holding an unused condom.

It reminds me of when I was in my mid-teens, dropping coins in the condom dispensing machine at one of only two women's clinics in Dublin. With the potential of giving in to the call of the wild, my friends and I wanted to be prepared. We knew the general population of Ireland were devoted Catholics and strictly followed the Catholic doctrines, and we were expected to behave accordingly. But becoming an unwed mother in that environment wasn't a wise choice, and we knew that sexually transmitted diseases and AIDS were running rampant. So, we made our choices.

At that time, our upbringing not only had limitations on age and marital status for entertaining intimate acts of love; the Catholic Church absolutely prohibited birth control with condoms. You didn't use them, you didn't talk about it, and you certainly didn't let anyone see you buy one. Sex before marriage was a sin and would make the Pope mad at you! So, I became the designated condom getter for the group brazen enough to access a condom vending machine placed just inside the door of one of the clinics.

It soon became a routine. Requests were placed, I would collect the money, and when needed, we would sneak off on our lunch break from our co-ed school to obtain as many condoms required to fill the requests. And I believed I was doing the right thing.

Often I'd hear my friends laughing outside to the endless sound of clink, clink, clink, from coins dropping through the metal slot, sometimes lasting more than twenty minutes. This act of friendship followed me later, and I would again be the condom supplier for a friend in Australia. She had an allergy to latex, which is believed to be caused from proteins in the liquid extracted from the banana tree. In the '90s, rubber condoms were difficult to find in the southern hemisphere, so I'd bring some back for her every time I traveled home. I knew I was not committing an illegal act, but when I returned to Australia with a year supply of rubber condoms, I felt as if I were transporting a banned substance, and my body language would betray me at the airport.

I wouldn't think twice about it until I checked in my luggage. Inevitably, someone in front of me would be pulled to the side with their suitcase to be opened in full view of the public. I watched the clothes and whatnots pile up on the table, and my brow would begin to percolate with sweat.

"Next!" a booming voice would call, bringing my attention back to the task at hand.

In front of me was a tall, muscle-bound, transportation safety agent, waving me up to the counter. The look on his face made it clear he wasn't there to be nice! I felt like I was walking the green mile, tugging the loaded bag behind me. As I wrestled the suitcase onto the conveyor, I was again startled by his voice and quickly passed my papers to the customs agent, pulling back quickly to hide the slight tremor of my shaking hand.

"Do you have anything to declare?" he asked.

"No sir!" I declared.

And with an exaggerated smile, I unconsciously quipped off small talk in attempt to distract from the contents of the suitcase. Heaven forbid my parents, or anyone else watch as the boxes of condoms are unloaded onto a table. Through the whole process, my eyes dart from side to side, waiting for the uniformed officials to flank me, waiting to be hauled off into a secure room for a possible strip search and waiting for the embarrassing speculations of why a young woman like me would be carrying such intimate booty into another country. Luckily, it never happened, but it would give me confidence to frequent sex shops a few years later. Not for sex toys or the like, but for pleasure of a different kind.

I had discovered that "kissing paint" was the closest I could ever get to tasting chocolate. It came in flavors of cherry chocolate, passion chocolate, etcetera. I wasn't going to use it to paint someone's body in the throes of passion, but to spread over my toast in the morning.

Improvisation works when you must avoid something you know without a doubt poses as a threat to your safety.

19

20 Minutes to Live

"Take a closer look at your reaction to reveal the pathway to healing. Look for what you avoid, physical symptoms, behavior, thoughts, emotions, and other responses associated with the event or final outcome. These are the signposts that point to the next step."

Journal Extract: Michelle Flanagan

Valentine's Day wasn't always a bed of roses and kissing paint as I recall my first really memorable kiss. It was one that I would never forget for many years to follow. The reader will understand why!

Already limited in our choices of dining options, my boyfriend and I decided to play it safe and dined at home before going to an English movie cinema to see Mel Gibson in his latest blockbuster *Brave Heart*. After all, we were living in a foreign country, and the opportunity to watch movies in English was a special treat.

There we were, cuddled together in the back row of a very small and dingy movie theatre, which at full capacity seated thirty young lovers, all silhouetted by the silver screen as excitement filled the air when the movie began. When the lights dimmed, my boyfriend leaned over and gave me a kiss: one that will be imprinted in my memory forever for the tingling sensations that it left behind. Inevitably, I was distracted from the opening scenes of the movie. Then I realized that my body was responding to something other than the kiss.

It was not responding to the happy warm and fuzzy feelings of love one would expect to feel on Valentine's Day. It was responding to a sense of impending doom as the warm sensations rushed through my body and set my lips on fire.

"Save yourself and get the hell out of there," my inner voice screamed, in a failed attempt to get me to do something about the pending danger evidenced by the ever-so-familiar sensations.

What a fool I was. I ignored the advice from my doctors to act immediately at the first signs of an allergic reaction. What was I doing just sitting there when it was obvious what was happening? I was confused because I hadn't eaten anything to bring this on, yet a sixth sense told me that my body was headed on a path of destruction and that the symptoms were only going to intensify until they led to death.

I slowly reached into my bag on the floor and slipped an antihistamine into my mouth, an action hidden from view to avoid any unnecessary attention. I knew from my past that a reaction took a lot longer than this to manifest. I still had time to reverse this, at least that's what I thought. Anything to avoid being an inconvenience! Maybe an antihistamine would fix the problem, and no one would be any wiser to the brief moment of anxiety I was now experiencing.

My usual response was never to ask for help until the symptoms were obvious to the naked eye and I couldn't hide them any more. My body was well and truly on its course of rejection, yet self pride stood in the way of me asking my boyfriend for any assistance when I clearly was beginning to need it.

I had passed my allergies off to him as nothing major if managed properly. I did this to avoid any chance of being rejected. I was happy to play Russian roulette with my life by staying silent. I would have done anything not to be a burden to him, so I pretended that I was just like everyone else, with just this little problem we needed to acknowledge—that it was really nothing. In truth, by not disclosing the full extent of what I knew about the problem was like tempting death.

I sat silently in my own despair and prayed that the antihistamines would work. My icy cold lemonade offered little solace to the burning metallic taste that had now traveled down the back of my throat. My stomach rumbled and the abdominal cramps started—shit! I needed a bathroom quick. I realized I was at the point of no return.

Still pretending that nothing was wrong, I gently whispered to my boyfriend that I would be back in a minute. Bewildered as to why I would leave so soon, he was fooled by my fake smile as I made my way to the end of the row, out the exit door, and hastily to the ladies' toilets.

A few minutes later, I was in real trouble, alone in the bathroom with vomit on my lips, uncontrollable diarrhea and a face that resembled something from a horror movie. I had giant swollen lips and eyes that looked like someone had taken me down a back alley and beaten me senseless. It was time to ask for help and risk being rejected. I returned to the movie theatre to save myself.

Interestingly enough, I didn't have to ask my boyfriend for help. All he had to do was look at me to know that we had an emergency on our hands. Our emergency action plan kicked in immediately, and like clockwork, we stepped out into the small lobby, assembled the syringe and needle, filled it with the prescribed amount of adrenaline and jabbed the needle sharply into my upper thigh muscle. Luckily I never left home without my syringe of adrenaline, knowing that one day it would save my life. That day had come and it was now! The handy adrenaline auto-injector used today wasn't available then, so we used a syringe.

I've often described the rush of adrenaline as feeling like having a million dollars backed on a horse and it's a photo finish. For a brief moment, time stands still before the heart races and every limb in your body shakes uncontrollably as the adrenaline rushes to every cell. I knew that the adrenaline impact would only buy me twenty minutes before the effects wore off, and I only had one shot. It was at that point that I remembered a doctor once telling me that the adrenaline should be administered even if it turned out to be a false alarm. "It will save your life," he told me. He couldn't stress enough that once it is administered, you must make your way to the nearest emergency room for medical treatment immediately. With only twenty minutes to live, we had to move quickly.

Without an ambulance in sight, we hailed down a taxi to take us to the nearest hospital. From memory it was a blessing in disguise that we were in Germany, as taxis were used as substitutes when an ambulance is unavailable.

"Can you go any faster?" my boyfriend said in German to the taxi driver as I quickly rolled down the back window and stuck my head out in an attempt to inhale as much icy February air as possible. The cold offered some relief to my burning throat as I choked amidst the wheezing and hives that engulfed my airways. It felt like I was in an elevator on a rapid descent. This is often the description used to describe a sudden drop in blood pressure.

By 8:25 p.m., all I wanted to do was fall asleep. It had only been twenty-five minutes from the time when we were cuddled together in the warm cinema, enjoying Valentine's Day. I slipped in and out of consciousness as I slowly drifted away.

"Stay with me," screamed my boyfriend in a voice filled with sheer panic. "We are at the hospital."

I tried to open my eyes. They were almost swollen shut, and I was gasping for breath as if someone had placed a ton of bricks on my chest.

Without question, I was wheeled straight into an emergency room cubicle, with the hospital personnel taking no time to investigate my medical history. Instead, my S.O.S bracelet was removed from my right wrist, revealing all inside. I was thankful that I wore one, now that I was in a state of shock and no longer realized what was happening. The bracelet was the only aid to fill in all the necessary gaps, as I couldn't be any help now.

"We are going to put you on an IV of steroids and give you an antihistamine," said the doctor. I remember feeling some sense of relief at that moment in the midst of the utter despair of the situation.

"We will periodically check your vitals; however, in the meantime, put this oxygen mask on to help you breathe," the nurse instructed.

The last thing I remember was the look of sheer helplessness and terror on my boyfriend's face. Even though I had trained him for this moment, it had taken its toll as he sat by my side, obviously in trauma. I had trained him what to do in an emergency; however, I had downplayed the severity of the reaction so that he would pass it off as nothing major. Despite still checking labels with me, etcetera, he wasn't prepared for the trauma or emotional impact of watching a loved one fight for her life. He had never even seen pictures of a reaction and was shocked when he saw the real thing. I had equipped him with skills that consisted of "What to do in the face of an emergency" and "An action plan in the event of", but I had never considered covering "How to deal with the psychological impact before, during, and after the event".

What a huge oversight on my part. He had witnessed my nightmare and clearly struggled to deal with the emotional impact of it.

After a few hours, it was evident that I was on the mend. My heart rate was back to normal, and I could breathe properly again. Despite a little swelling around my face and slight nausea, I knew that it was time to speak with the doctor.

"We can see from your case history that you have been allergic to peanuts and shellfish most of your life. Did you have anything to eat over the last few hours that may have brought on an allergic reaction?" the doctor asked.

"No, I didn't," I responded, confused. I had wracked my brains, unable to find any obvious cause. He then asked me to back track to what I was doing just before I started to notice the symptoms.

"We were in the cinema. I made sure that I didn't eat anything while I was there because I really wanted to have a memorable Valentine's Day." I nervously laughed, thinking to myself that today was definitely memorable.

"We kissed just before the movie started, but we have always been very careful, haven't we?" I directed my question to my boyfriend. The doctor turned to my boyfriend and asked him, "Did you eat any peanuts or shellfish today?"

"Oh, shit! I had peanuts during my lunch break, but we've had dinner and a few drinks since then. I kissed Michelle at about 8:00 p.m., which was hours after I ate them," my boyfriend responded in disbelief. The blood drained from his face as he realized that he was the likely catalyst of this reaction.

The doctor proceeded to explain what had just happened.

"Michelle, you just had another Anaphylactic allergic reaction."

Duh! As if I didn't know already, I thought.

"In your case, following the kiss, it began with a tingling sensation, itching, and a metallic taste in your mouth, stomach cramps, vomiting, diarrhea, swelling of the mouth and eyes, difficulty breathing, hives, and a sudden drop in blood pressure.

"You are a very lucky girl. The adrenaline saved your life. It gave you just enough time to get here for lifesaving treatment. Without it, you might not be with us. You shall be staying in hospital tonight so that we can monitor you because of the possibility of having a repeat reaction.

"You must be more vigilant in the future to avoid peanuts, as your sensitivity to the allergen has obviously increased. We shall put you on a course of steroids for a week, and I would like you to make an appointment with our allergy clinic to review your medical history by doing more allergy tests."

Even though I had already lived a life avoiding peanuts, nothing could have prepared me for this. This reaction was pretty full on. How could it possibly be any worse the next time?

I was told to take some time to let everything sink in and come back the following week with any questions that I might have. It was time for my boyfriend to go home, and he approached me for a kiss goodbye. He stopped as he got closer and thought for a second.

"Not tonight, my dear," he said, smiling as he blew me a kiss across the room. "I can't believe that I nearly gave you the 'Kiss of Death' on Valentine's Day!"

I smiled and blew a kiss right back at him, knowing deep down that tonight might have changed our relationship forever.

It did and it didn't.

We actually stayed together for another few years, but he became over-protective and pedantic about every little thing, driven by fear that I'd react again. (I did, two times after this incident, during one of which I required CPR.) This indeed would affect our relationship in profound ways, eventually ending it.

But that didn't matter right now, as there is never a day you are more thankful for than the day you almost die yet manage to live.

When I look back now, I never talked with him about this incident or the others that followed. If they came up in conversation, I brushed them off. The incidents had always been about me, I thought; I encountered the reaction; I was the one suffering; I would deal with it on my own to protect others from the emotional impact. I never once realized that other people around me were also affected. They wanted to help and had accepted my imperfections. I hadn't. His need to talk about it was his way of dealing with his own trauma and fears.

Becoming over-protective was his way of keeping me safe and out of harm's way. But I interpreted it as someone trying to control me. But wasn't maintaining some control the same—part of efforts to keep me safe? It was imbalanced only because my side lacked the ability to share, to work on solutions together, to trust the other. I felt boxed in, as if by large balls of cotton wool that were trying to smother me even more than my life was already structured. The invisible prison walls were closing in, and I had to break free.

In hindsight, maybe if I had stopped for a moment and listened to him, rather than being a martyr dealing with everything on my own, things might have turned out differently between us.

20
The Sound Of Silence

"If I were not a physicist, I would probably be
a musician. I often think in music. I live my
daydreams in music. I see my life in terms of
music...I get most joy in life out of music."

Albert Einstein

"You never listen," I recall the words often said to me
while I was growing up. Maybe there was some truth
behind this. When the inside of my nose tingled, a
sneeze was coming. If it was my bladder, I had to pee.
When my lips tingled, this was a sure sign of an
impending allergic reaction. But I didn't listen to my
body's messaging system until I had no choice about it.
While out in the most unlikely of places, the reason why
this was so rang as clear as a bell on a summer's day.

It was a night when my local pub overflowed with audacious
performers and unheard whispers of internal dialogue: "Maybe I'll be
discovered", "I can do better than him", "Oh my nerves...what if I get
stage-fright?", "or worse still...what if I pee on myself?" pre-nerve
utterances of hidden voices waiting their turn to be discovered.

It was Karaoke night—a night when anything could happen.
Karaoke meaning "kara" (empty) and "okestura" (orchestra); a night
when the brave sing, the talented shine, and loyal onlookers listen or
cringe. However, they applaud their friend regardless—some sing, not
in perfect harmony or even in tune, but with heart.

"Pretend you are singing," I recall a nun telling her pre-selected
inept group of six year old singers in preparation for our First Holy
Communion. "God has gifted your friend with the voice of
angels...not you," were her words to me. "Just open and close your
mouth...don't let the sound out...Mum and Dad will hear their angel
sing anyway," preached the nun. This was her shaming device during

hymn practice. How young and naive I was to imprint her every word as true and be haunted by it in years to come. But I was only six years old.

This was the nun's chance to shine at the Convent school's biggest annual event. She would be the hymn teacher behind our righteous and holy performance. Whatever her intention, "The Art of Mime" imprinted my psyche—I would only lip synch so as to keep my "discordant" voice from ruining her big moment.

Despite having to turn on the mute button during the day at practice, the singer within broke free from its cage every night, like a bird. Without fail I'd launch into chorus at bedtime to a private audience—my sister. Instead of rose petals and flowers as recognition for my budding performance of "Ave Maria" or the latest hymn from practice, my singing would be met with flying pillows, teddy bears, dolls, or whatever else could be propelled towards my direction.

"Michelle...will you be quiet! I can't sleep," stressed my seven year old sister as a teddy bounced off the wall beside me. "I will tell Mum if you don't shut up."

Irritation and impatience was heard in my idol's voice from the bed next to me. I had learned at school as a six year old that it was not cool to sing out loud. Mime! Whatever you do, don't let out any sound. That is for the gifted. I'm sure my sister would have been happier if I had listened.

That year the invisible belt tightened even further around my voice box, trapping the angel's lullaby within.

I remember first hearing about Karaoke night and cringing for fear I'd fold under the pressure to sing. I decided to go. I'd stand my ground. I'd just listen.

"I'd like to welcome our next performer...Jack...he is going to sing 'A Different Beat' by Boyzone...a band from Ireland," sounded the speakers.

Immediately my ears perked up. This was my brother's favorite song. Every time I heard this particular song, especially while away from my family, the beat always unlocked a special place in my heart, releasing a cascade of memories of home, flooding my arteries with warm and fuzzy feelings that flowed to my roots, to my bones.

"Not this time," I said to myself disappointed as soon as Jack began to release his unique take on the song. "Help!" cried my ears. If only he knew how to follow the advice of my hymn teacher, I thought wistfully. I automatically stopped listening as if an internal switch had tripped, sending a warning to trance out.

"The pitch...someone please lower the pitch...it's making me dizzy...turn the volume down...switch off...please switch off this awful noise."

His voice chiseled away at my soul as it killed any sentiment or sense of belonging attached to this song. This once welcome sound was rejected—the inner jury had come in.

Yet all incoming sound had been muted. I wondered why.

I had unknowingly ventured into the recesses of my past.

My mind began to play back a hymn I had once heard—it was a sound from heaven. Then it led me to a distant world switched off to the outside world—when the incoming orchestra of sound was "kara" (empty).

I was eighteen months old and despite not remembering much about this time, Mum filled in the blanks.

"   ," said Mum, standing over the threshold of the living room door. "   ," she repeated as I sat quietly on the carpet, totally submerged in self-amusement in the corner of the living room. Contentment was ushered into my baby space, scribbling my masterpieces on paper with crayon—or anything else I could find in the vicinity.

"   ," she said again waiting in anticipation for my first utterance. I had reached an age of firsts; first to string two words together besides "Mummy" and "Daddy"; first to recognize objects upon hearing their names; first to follow commands when spoken to; first to walk upright with balance and confidence; first to communicate with the outside world; and first to gain an energetic connection with the digestive system, personal power, and life direction.

"   ," was uttered in a louder and even more piercing tone. Still no response! More was said; she was increasing her pitch as she got closer—now she was flapping her arms about like a penguin trying to take flight. But she would soon realize even the loudest claps or foot stomps elicited little or no response. She instinctively knew something about this didn't seem black and white—its truth held shades of gray.

"   ," she said again, waving a cup in front of my eyes.

"Ah! Food," I thought, eventually awarding her presence with a huge innocent bright smile. But this time Mummy's face expressed a kind of unfamiliarity about it, something I hadn't seen before—distress and worry. Her endless cries of my name had been lost in a muffled silence. At eighteen months there was no way I could know that the muffled world I lived was not normal. Unresponsiveness alerted her that something wasn't quite right. This would mark the first of many visits to doctors thereafter.

"From what I can tell, Michelle has a build-up of fluid behind both eardrums," said the specialist at Dublin's Children's Hospital. "The ear canal in babies and young children under the age of five is still narrow, so a build up or blockage of fluid is sometimes likely."

"Ear wax?" Mum asked

"During a child's growth there may be times when ear wax production levels are higher than normal, which causes the wax to leak out of the ear. If there is no fever, no complaints of earache, and the wax is without a smelly odor…then this is probably just excessive ear wax. But when these symptoms are present, this may indicate an infection, inflammation and/or a blockage of thick, sticky-like fluid in the middle ear chamber (*otitis media*) that has leaked into the ear canal."

"Yes she has a temperature," the doctor replied confirming an infection.

"Can she hear anything?" asked mum concerned.

"She can hear, but sound may be muffled. This glue-like fluid can impair the vibration of the small bones in the ear cavity that transmits sound. This is why she may not respond to quiet sound, might seem inattentive, or might not turn around when you walk up behind her," he replied.

"An infection such as a cold or flu can contribute to mucus blockage in the tubes—the passage between the middle ear and the pharynx," he said pointing to the part of the throat situated immediately behind the mouth and nasal cavity to indicate the pharynx.

"How is this treated?" Mum asked.

"Generally the fluid clears up on its own. There is an operation where 'grommets' or little plastic tubes can be inserted into the ear canal to allow air to flow and the fluid to drain…This treatment is relatively new so I'd like to hold off until Michelle is a bit older…and to see if the fluid clears up on its own. Put this oil in both ears at night before she goes to sleep…it should help to alleviate some of the blockage and hopefully clear it," he said.

Every night for two years thereafter, my tears flooded the bedroom as mum poured warm oil into both ears. It was a time when cotton balls plugged my nightly world into total silence. Surpassing the earache, comfort came from my mum gently stroking my hair and knowing my sister Paula was close by. Fear and anxiety began to write a bedtime story into my internal guidebook, the early stage of problems later.

Despite the trauma at night, during the day I amused myself for hours painting infant masterpieces. My body's adaptation abilities had flourished, replacing the hearing loss with a heightened visual sense. Color became my world. The left hemisphere of the brain that is considered the seat of language was less active, and the right hemisphere became skilled at understanding spatial, visual and motor information, and took control. Communication came as pictures and hues rather than listened to or spoken words. With one sense down, the body's adaptive nature remapped another sense to accommodate— in my case, sight.

Sound clarity and balance finally arrived at the age of three and a half—the insertion of "grommets" was a success. But the operation would become two-fold. Due to repeatedly inflamed tonsils (tonsillitis), they were removed. My tonsils, the first line of defense against ingested or inhaled foreign pathogens, were all but gaping holes. I would leave the hospital with the gift of sound but also with weakened defenses in the mouth and nose regions. Air, water, and food—crucial needs for survival—now posed as threats or were even dangerous, especially now that I had entered the age of food exploration.

A surgeon had removed a problem area that could not possibly have come into existence without a cause. It had inflamed in response to a cause, and the inflammation and response were very likely to come back because the cause was left untouched. Had the fluid build-up in the nasal and throat cavity been initially misconstrued as a cold? But was it instead a first line of defense against something ingested, inhaled, or deficient—unnoticed? Tonsils have a privileged situation in the immune system in that they are in touch with the environment. With defenses down, my body now had extra work. Left to adapt, it did what it always did: that is, it learned from the conditions of the environment. But now the immune system without the help of the tonsils was blinded to environmental factors. And the ears, now relieved of the blockage, didn't have sound's great reference book written yet. The only sense that memorized new molecules like the immune system was the nose—the olfactory system.

Was the cause of the inflammation still in the environment? What was my body to do except do its best in spite of the fact that part of its defense walls had been compromised. If the enemy was still present, where and when would it attack again? Defense had no choice but to turn to olfactory for help as it regrouped. With a massive increase in the use of chemicals such as pesticides on fresh fruit and in household cleaning products, and other toxins and synthetic proteins in the environment, it was only a matter of time before the defenses would be alerted to act again—this time with an untrained, inexperienced defense team now wearing blinkers.

"What will you be when you grow up?" asked an uncle when I was about five years old.

"I am going to Art College, of course." That was always my reply, and I was puzzled as to why every big person asked the same questions when all my drawings made that abundantly clear.

I began school not long after the operation, as if thrown in at the deep end to catch up on language and speech development. Even though I was still young memories of my elocution teacher, Mrs. Cobalt, still ring as clear as bells in my mind. The significance of this teacher wouldn't become apparent until I started to look at my childhood with fresh eyes.

Mrs. Cobalt came to the school once a week to teach us how to speak properly. Considering my situation, I found the timing of her arrival into my life uncanny. Rain or shine, she always wore a leopard printed coat. She could be seen for miles, distinguished by a false animal hide with which she was covered from head to toe, complete with a long trailing blue scarf tightly wrapped around her neck. Her knee-length bright-colored socks added more mystery to her oddness. Her strange and eccentric sense of attire stuck in my mind—any child would swear that she came from a cartoon. She oozed energy and mystery, something I will never forget.

Then there was her pet.

Albert.

Always in hand was her leather lead, the kind you'd use for a medium size dog. It was bright and intriguing, just like her.

"It's to keep him tame," she'd say referring to Albert.

Her pet leopard.

I never consciously saw Albert but my imagination did.

"Close the windows, girls...I don't want him to jump out," were her instructions. We always followed her instructions to the letter for fear Albert would run away.

"Julie, it's your turn to get Albert a drink." She would pick a child at random, handing over the famous blue dish to be filled with water.

"Leave it on the floor next to him," Mrs. Cobalt directed. I can still remember feeling a bit unprotected and vulnerable every time it was my turn, hoping I got the location right.

But she told us that he was a model pet—always on his best behavior. I believed her. He never once stirred from the corner of the classroom! There was no cause for alarm while she conducted the lesson. But it still didn't stop me from listening for a noise, sometimes convinced I heard a roar or a growl from the corner. A burp even! My imagination probably manufactured these sounds.

Albert was real in my childhood world.

What reason would I have not to hear him?

"Okay, girls...let's begin," she'd say.

"I want you to place a finger on either side of your mouth and squeeze when you say these words."

"Hooow...Noooow...Brooown...Cooow," she said, while demonstrating, squeezing her fingers together.

"Squeeze those fingers together when you say "OW" girls...put emphasis on this OW sound.

"Great...let's do it again...repeat after me...how...now...brown... cow," she said as the class erupted into a weird and wonderful rhythm. Once it was perfected, we moved onto the next lesson.

"Peter Piper picked a...," we'd chant, laughing when the words came out all jumbled—the times when we couldn't seem to get our tongues around the vocals. Laughter refreshed the airways and cleansed the soul.

"Okay, can everyone stand up, please, and start shaking your shoulders...now roll them...loosen them up...wriggle them up and down...and while you move them around I want you to start humming…wriggle about…even louder…I want to hear the room hum like a bee," she instructed as the classroom erupted into an energetic buzz of movement and sound. I will never forget it. Who would have thought that learning how to speak could be so much fun?

As the weeks progressed, so too did various types of exercises; rolling our heads back and forth, around in circles, sideways, front and back, in opposing directions, singing, humming, yawning—various methods to release tension in and around the voice box.

The principal always knew when Mrs. Cobalt was in the school. Sounds of children humming like bees to honey on a spring day echoed throughout the corridors. Sighs of relief and cheers were heard through laughter.

My main teacher, Miss Arden, taught language, math, reading, writing, and general subjects for most five and six year olds. Hymns and prayers in preparation for my first Holy Communion had been added to the usual curriculum. This was Sr. Ann's domain.

If asked to use one word that best described my memory of Miss Arden it would be "cold". I can still recall feeling the freshness of the winter day, breezing through large Georgian style windows left wide open to flush out the stuffy warm classroom air.

"Germs, germ, germs…." Miss Arden often used to say. "They will make you sick," said, her words triggering a memory that had once been written in the internal survival guidebook so long ago. Retrieved like a foghorn through dense fog, sounding loud and clear. My stomach gurgled at the idea of being sick.

"Open all the windows wide." I can still recall feeling the burst of winter enter the cozy classroom air.

"I am cold," was a common child's cry, often ignored. Germ warfare and eradication often took precedence.

On really cold days the windows were shut tight. But they were open if it was a lesson involving twenty or so young mouths all speaking at the same time. Then the freshness of the outside air was felt by all. It was common practice to open the windows as soon as Mrs. Cobalt had left the room.

I often thought this was to let Albert out.

"Germs are most active when you sneeze, cough, or splutter…especially when you have a cold…" Miss Arden's haunting words flash to mind.

"As soon as you feel a sneeze coming...hold your nose...," she'd repeat like a broken record, her intensity heightened during the cold and flu season. If you coughed, you covered your mouth. Either way, I had learned to hold my breath, not to breathe, to invert. This was a contradiction of the lessons taught by Mrs. Cobalt.

"I will give you twenty lines to write on the board if you don't," were her punishing words. The thought "I must not spread my germs," still rings alarm bells in my memory center.

But as soon as the windows were opened, a fit of sneezing and coughing always began. I couldn't understand why, except that our written lines put the fear of God into us, a subliminal message in full view on the blackboard for all to see. Terrified to sneeze or cough for fear I'd be punished, I'd hold it in, fearing that blood would start to flow, my ears would pop and stop hearing, or my throat would gag and tighten. I didn't realize that I had learned that sneezing was bad. Even hearing someone else sneeze alerted my body to hold in air, to trigger sorrow for those awaiting punishment, inducing a state of worry that the next time the punishment might be mine.

Miss Arden had unknowingly taught me to hold my nose and mouth every time a tickle sensation was felt inside the nasal passage, a retrained defense mechanism that would carry into adulthood. Through adaptation the body redirected the powerful blasts of air out via my ears. The sneeze was supposed to be an immune defense to expel foreign particles from my airways. But now the blast was leaving my ear passages like dynamite. But what of the foreign particles my body had been trying to expel? Where did they go? And what if my defense had been relying more on my nose—adaptation since the loss of the tonsils? Thus children are often programmed to have health issues, even by well-meaning teachers.

Sr. Ann got her recognition for our first Holy Communion performance, and my parents would hear my silent angel lullaby.

I wouldn't find "my song" until high school and even then it would hide from me. Miss Thomson, my music teacher, entered my life when I was in my early to mid teens. She was young, probably in her late twenties at the time, and she was rumored to have a drinking problem. The other girls had commented on occasion about her beer breath just after lunch. This exaggeration would prove to be nothing more than the work of those who were frightened into believing alcohol was wrong; exaggerating was the perfect way to get those who were curious about the topic to listen.

Music from the '70s and '80s was the trend at the time, the sound vibrating from the radio. I often cranked up the volume to watch the stereo speakers vibrate in rhythm to the song that was playing at the time. Music wasn't just entertainment; it touched me. It helped to heal growing pains. My body felt it, like a tuning fork of sound waves vibrating in my soul.

Miss Thomson would expand my world with the introduction to classical music. But for me, there was nothing more boring than a class of about thirty five teenage girls spending forty minutes at a time listening to old vinyl records: Bach, Beethoven, Mozart; you name it, we listened to it. This music was for the oldies. This class was a snooze fest. I didn't get it then. I can still remember yawning while resting my head on a makeshift pillow, my folded arms. I pretended to listen but instead I was catching some Zs. Classical music almost always put me to sleep.

Some times we sang, while other times we'd learn how to read music—the tone, beat, vibration, notes, music history, and so on. I wouldn't realize the significance of this class until on my path of unfoldment.

"DO, RE, MI, FA, SO, LA, TI..." the common sounds echoed through the corridors as we practiced our musical scales. It was a far cry from the humming and chanting heard many years before when we were small. The angels had turned up the volume. Sound once lost in time as echoes would eventually find their way back to me.

On my path of healing later on, I can still recall my first class on the state of being fully aware of the present—the art of meditation. A group of us sat in what can best be described as a calm and peaceful environment; gentle music was playing in the background; soft lighting relaxed the senses; and the tone of the teacher's voice radiated peace.

As usual, upon arrival, anxiety scanned the room for evidence of risk: incense, oil burners, oils, specific aromatic candles, or any edibles—anything that posed as a potential cause of an allergic incident.

The coast was clear.

The school had listened to me by adhering to my specific set of safety requirements. Uneasiness still remained but the volume was lower.

"Meditation is easy to learn but the effects are beyond imagination—powerful," she said in a slow rhythmic lull. "It has been known to release energy within the body, which the body uses to heal."

I liked to be busy, always on the go. My first impression of meditation was like classical music—if it put me asleep or slowed me down in any way, I wasn't interested. But with a health crisis literally on my doorstep, this attitude was a luxury I couldn't afford.

A little willingness to change my perception was all it took to give meditation a go. Little did I know that I was about to learn something I had never been told about sound before.

This would become very significant.

"What is that lovely background music," I can still recall asking the teacher during a break. As always, I stayed in the course room during breaks, afraid to mingle where food was present, especially amidst an unfamiliar group.

"It's one of the last remaining ancient Gregorian chants. This one is called 'The Hymn to St. John the Baptist'," she replied, smiling, and handing me the CD cover.

I was noticeably really relaxed—a far cry from my anxious state earlier. Strangely, this sound calmed me down.

"What do you mean by 'last remaining'?" I asked, like a detective on a mission to reclaim what my ears may have once lost.

"Do you know the musical scale "DO, RE, MI…?" she asked. I nodded, telling her about my school days.

"I learned it at school. I didn't obsess about music like my school friends but I did like learning how to read and write music. I used to write my own lyrics when I was a teen. But so did some of my friends. I used to practice the musical scales on the piano every Saturday morning. It was just a passing phase, though. I believe the repetition nearly drove my sister mad," I said with a snigger.

"Every sound is different because it has its own unique vibration; a bell ringing, a dog's bark, a sneeze, a musical note, your computer, street traffic, a siren, your voice and so on," she began to explain.

We were interrupted by the sound of a plane as it passed outside— an alien sound in this tranquil place.

"Like that plane," I said.

She nodded.

I thought of how my voice had changed to a slight stutter after the traumatic incident in Munich. How my voice changed during an anaphylactic reaction. How it altered when I had a cold. It was the vibration that had changed—the sound waves.

"Sound can be very powerful—it can literally transform and heal you. It doesn't matter if you can hear the sound or not. But the musical scale has been altered over time and now misses vast healing capabilities the ancient scale had—found in Gregorian chants like this one," she said pointing to the stereo speaker.

"The 'original solfeggio frequencies' as they are called contain special tones or sound wave frequencies believed to penetrate deep in the subconscious to promote healing. But, sadly, a number of these ancient chants were lost around 1050 A.D. There is only a few remaining," she explained.

"This is exactly what I came here to learn," I thought, asking her to tell me more about sound with its miraculous healing powers.

"The Solfeggio frequencies contain six pure notes: UT, RE, MI, FA, SO, LA.' These notes were altered by the Catholic Church some time around 590 A.D., which eventually gave rise to the modern scale DO, RE, MI, FA, SO, LA. The seventh note 'TI' was added later. So the modern musical scale is slightly out of sync and does not hold the same healing and transformational properties as the ancient scale did."

"Oh! I can really feel different sensations firing off around my body listening to this hymn," I laughed and giggled, curious to know more. "Is this normal?" I couldn't believe that the sound I was hearing was tickling certain parts of my body. That it could have such an impact! If I wasn't feeling the effects I would have never believed it.

"The hymn you are listening to contains all six notes that make the ancient scale. Each note is associated with a certain part of your body, a specific color, a musical note, and their corresponding frequency number." My face was blank.

"Let me explain: middle C of the original solfeggio scale is related to the 528 Hz frequency (528 sound waves per second), and middle C as we know it today vibrates at 512 Hz. The 528 Hz frequency corresponds with 'MI' on the musical scale, the color green, and is associated with the heart and immune system. It is called the 'miracle' frequency known to regenerate the body and repair DNA," she concluded.

"Wow," I said. My mouth was wide open in disbelief. If sound could have such an effect on the body, then what effect does manmade sound have on my body? I wondered. The hunter-gatherers wouldn't have felt the same sound vibrations we have today; sound emanating from a passing plane, a car, a siren, a computer, a ticking clock, electricity, a humming fridge—modern sounds created due to technological advancements, particularly over the last forty years. Nor did they have the diseases we face today. Nor did they make the same language sounds—most ancient languages have since been lost in time.

Had I just found the gene reset button?

I replayed what I had just heard in my mind. I was excited.

My body is a walking orchestra of different sounds: a sigh, burp, cough, gurgle, fart, sniff, swallow, roar, growl, and so on. In essence these various noises are just different vibrations or frequencies. The vibration of the musical notes physically corresponds to the part of the body vibrating at the same frequency. No wonder I could literally feel certain songs. No wonder I was affected by what I was telling myself or that a change in someone's tone and even what I was saying was in essence an alteration to the vibration or frequency my body was transmitting or receiving.

No wonder my body still functioned regardless of whether I could hear or not. It read and felt vibrations—without vibration it couldn't survive. Is this how my cells communicate, I wondered—did they pick up signals from the unique vibrational fingerprints throughout the system? If the frequency or vibration changed or altered in any area, then the information or message could get lost, distorted or misinterpreted, couldn't it?.

I had learned that certain immune cells responded to specific signals emanating from fungus spores, bacteria, viruses, etcetera. Could a change in vibration explain how the defense system could have misinterpreted something harmless to be an enemy? If this were true, then I'd be more in control if I learned how to decipher and understand how different vibrations or frequencies could impact me. If different frequencies altered the biochemistry and physiology of the body—invisible waves that link internal and external environments—

had I found missing puzzle pieces? And had I found it only because silence had played such a major role in my life?

My mission was to find these Solfeggio frequencies, to learn more about what notes or frequencies corresponded with what bodily parts. What if I self-prescribed daily sound therapy to the areas I felt were in desperate need of repair or retuning? Could listening to Solfeggio frequencies help to reset the gene switchboard? I believed it could.

This class gave me an idea.

An experiment!

Surely if the frequency or vibration changed in my voice box, so too would the sound of my voice.

Over the next few weeks I hummed, rolled my neck around, jiggled my shoulders about, learned to take a breath, listened to frequencies, and sang with sound. I practiced daily bioenergetics, a specific type of exercise that uses a combination of vibration, sound, and movement to release blocked energy flow. I learned to listen to what others were saying, but also what I had been saying to myself.

That day I would meditate for the very first time.

I still meditate today.

The experiment's testing day had arrived.

"Our next performer to the stage is Michelle...she is going to sing...,"continued the announcer as I positioned myself in front of my loyal onlookers.

The pub was packed, more so than ever before.

My hands shook with nerves but that was okay.

My energy was flowing. I picked up the microphone and began to sing to a different beat like I never had before.

My friends had never heard me sing; in fact, neither had I.

I finally understood Jack, he gave heart.

My heart and soul gave it all, best described as nothing less than awesome. The last note played to deafening applause.

Jack, in the crowd, clapped too.

"We'd like to add you as one of our contestants for the pub's next Karaoke Idol competition," the commentator said while handing me the registration details.

I felt humbled and surprised.

My experiment had been more of a success than I had thought it would be. It was not because I had been invited to enter the Karaoke competition, but because my own singing idol had come out of her silence. Tonight, for the first time, the waves blew freely in the wind and the butterfly was released to sing an angel's lullaby.

21
Déjà Vu Up Close & Personal
"How you react is dictated by how nature has shaped you and by what you have learned from experience."
Journal Extract: Michelle Flanagan

Like a cat with multiple lives, by now I had encountered way too many near-death experiences for any one lifetime. And memory had no mercy—the imprints of these events lay waiting as constant reminders of my situation. Unusual circumstances always stood out, moments I now believe my inner intelligence purposely brought forward as an attempt to teach my conscious mind something. But I ignored or didn't recognize the lessons so as to keep the peace—downgrading these experiences as normal. They were anything but. And no matter what I did, the fighter always persisted; each message got louder. Finding resolution depended on discovering the right buttons to turn the volume down.

The sirens could be heard in the distance, a welcome sound for the onlookers at the scene of this unpredicted incident of shock. I was one of them. I was almost like an observer of my own fate as my body lay still and internally swollen; the ounce of fight left within almost expired. Sirens were a common sound in this particular part of Sydney. Drug overdoses and domestic violence were not unusual in this neighborhood, but the rent was cheap.

It was my first Australian summer: long clammy nights and hot days—the total opposite of the blizzard I had just left behind in Washington. One commonality prevailed—this city would also catch me up close and personal, not once but twice. In Sydney, despite it being such a different place on the planet than I was used to, brought many déjà vu experiences. A sense of déjà vu permeated the people, the food, the culture, and even some of my social activities. Playing a game of pool or billiards, meeting friends for a drink on a lazy Sunday afternoon, or going for a stroll in the park had commonality with all my life experiences. It didn't matter where I was on the globe, allergy management was always at the forefront—I did everything within my power to avoid a traumatic incident.

"Somebody please help!" my boyfriend cried in a panic-stricken voice as he fumbled to assemble a syringe with just the right amount of epinephrine (adrenaline). If he didn't, I was dead. Luckily, he had now joined me in Sydney, making the journey as I had from Munich a couple of months before. By now he had learned how to administer the adrenaline since our almost fatal kiss on Valentine's Day only two and a half years prior. I still didn't have the adrenaline auto-injector then, so learning how to assemble the syringe's bits and pieces, coupled with getting the right measure of adrenaline were essential to saving my life. But the addition of high stress would prove this task extremely difficult. He had only ever practiced on injecting oranges. Performance anxiety had set in—he knew that without epinephrine my life hung in the balance.

"Please help!" he cried even louder, bending over my limp body, slumped like a rag doll on the doorstep of an inner city pub. The late afternoon sun shone on my already reddened face, the shadow as the sun passed over wasn't the only thing engulfing me.

Despite the distressing situation, people continued to walk past us, to and fro, back and forth, regardless of his desperate cries for help. This emergency to them was just smoke—an incident to wave from their internal memory banks as unrelated to them. It was an unimportant event in a drug-stricken neighborhood where substance abuse was rife. Did they think I was a junky in need of a fix? That my plight had been self-inflicted and therefore I deserved my sentence? Or were they just numb to this common neighborhood sight, passing the buck to trained professionals, the paramedics, leaving them to deal with me?

This unhelpful behavior based upon their judgment had given me a death sentence. It was now clear that any plea for help would be ignored. I'm sure if they knew the circumstances, they would stop to offer help. But they didn't. They kept walking. They didn't know the situation. How could they? This particular allergic reaction swelled internally. The usual inflammation wasn't visible. But even if it was, in this part of town facial swelling may have been misconstrued as domestic violence. To any passer-by, the first impression of an unconscious body limp on the sidewalk—on a pub's doorstep, no less, the common hangout for a drunk—would not cause undue alarm. To make things worse, this almost lifeless body came with a distressed partner holding a syringe in hand for all to see.

We had chosen to move to this dodgy neighborhood with a couple of friends only a few months before. The rent for a large house was cheap. I hadn't once given any thought to how my place of residence could be detrimental to my fate. And I couldn't now.

"How could so many people not see me?" asked my soul, looking on. It was now watching over me, in an out-of-body experience. "They walk as if I am not here."

"Hello, I need help," my soul frantically moved toward each and every passer-by, yelling in their ears in hope that someone would respond. But they couldn't or didn't want to hear. Instead they carried on about their business as if my body was invisible. In their eyes, I was.

"Wow, that guy is staring right at me, yet he whistles past as if nothing is happening...even the passing traffic are going slower...desperate to get a peak to satisfy their curiosity. They put their trust in someone else to handle this...they believe it's not their problem."

"Can you not see that my boyfriend is trying to save my life...that he needs your help?" my internal essence strained to reach them. "Is it fear that binds you to the side lines? That prevents you from lending a hand? That stops you from acting? Or is it ignorance that keeps you away from what you don't know? Yet for a brief moment curiosity engages you. It gives you a choice point, a moment to choose to engage in this situation or not."

The smell of rubber from the passing tires was almost sickening—my sense of smell had turned up the volume to the maximum. I could now taste other people's ignorance and fear in my mouth. But what could I do now? I lay helpless in the shadows.

"Call an ambulance," yelled my boyfriend through a crack in the doorway of the pub. He did this to alert the patrons to the commotion on their doorstep—his sense of urgency told them there wasn't much time.

"I can't do this," he said to the local patrons now gathering on the street. "Help me! She is having an allergic reaction to food."

Drops of sweat from his brow fell on my cheek. My unconscious could taste salt as it waited to be jolted from this paralyzing bind. I couldn't move. My body had gone into total disarray as internal programming had clashed the systems.

A substantial group had now gathered. Whether I liked it or not, I was center stage. There were no curtains to hide behind. This demon was now under the spotlight, shining in all its glory. Unconscious, I still labored for air. It felt as if a ten ton truck had parked on my chest.

"She's having an allergic reaction...I have to administer this," my boyfriend frantically repeated, pointing to the syringe. His nervous energy begged for someone to help. To listen! To take action!

"Here, let me do it," said an earthly angel from the crowd as he motioned for the syringe. "My mum is a diabetic," said a slight, slightly balding man who had stepped forward, indicating that he wasn't a drug user. "Just tell me where to administer the injection."

By now my boyfriend was speechless. Anxiety had consumed him. His energy had deflated. This angel had given him a moment to recharge, to take a breath, to recompose himself.

"My name is Paul," the man said, gesturing a quick handshake in an attempt to dissolve some of the panic infecting the air. His head moved closer to catch the sound of my breath. The smell of stale tobacco entered my nostrils but that didn't matter—I was breathing.

"We need to lower her jeans slightly," instructed my boyfriend. "The injection needs to go into the upper thigh muscle...I want to make sure that the fabric doesn't get in the way," he said, opening my top button and lowering the zip.

Any embarrassment would be swept on a tide to oblivion. A red face is irrelevant when survival takes over. Actually, whenever you encounter a perceived threat to survival—a major upheaval, a life-threatening event, intense stress, or a gradual build up toward a crisis point, something very interesting happens. It's as if the body splits in two. One part fires shockwaves of thunder, as if screaming at you to fight or run away; and the other whispers of temporary reprieve and slows down. In a moment of sheer terror and confusion, they may clash so as to put your systems into paralysis. The familiar idea of reality is pillaged and reconstructed in a way that profoundly alters you.

Sometimes you are left bound up in a hostage take-over by the screamer, blinded by pain and turmoil, and often robbed of peace.

It didn't matter that we had moved into this neighborhood only a few weeks before—that our clothes were still unpacked and that household chores such as laundry had been mounting. Nor did it matter that my underpants on show today were the most unflattering pair ever seen in the world. They would almost certainly win first prize in a lingerie contest for grannies. They had been written about in Bridget Jones' Diary—they were giant, flesh-colored spandex designed to engulf the lower abdomen to compress and conceal the bulges, the bumps, and the excess flab. A friend had given them to me as a joke when I turned twenty-five. The intention had never been to wear them, or to be caught dead in them. Why I was even wearing them in the first place baffled me. That didn't matter now. But it would later.

When life hangs in the balance, there is no room for ego. Blushing generally comes in the aftermath if you meet your audience again. Pride didn't matter now—my life did.

"Move away and give her some air," an onlooker directed the growing numbers trying to catch a glimpse of the action.

Traffic had nearly come to a standstill—all the drivers of the cars heading in both directions had their eyes wide open.

"The ambulance is on the way," said one of the bar staff, sticking his head out of the pub entrance. "It should be here any minute."

People were now lending a hand. They had seen my red flag. This sudden change in willingness to assist surprised me.

"Inject her here!" said my boyfriend. "Don't get the vein…it has to be injected into the muscle," his tone shifted to emphasize this very important fact.

So much had happened in such a short space of time. Knowledge of what may have triggered this reaction was irrelevant. Getting to the hospital was the only important thing.

"Is this my time?" asked my ghostly self, standing over my own body confused. I felt detached and bewildered as if I had just dropped one hundred flights of stairs in an elevator. I was sinking fast. Thoughts of my beginning and now my possible end flashed holographic images into my mind's eye. Imprinted memories of the circle of life I had lived were flashing before me.

Had I come full circle?

Was this the end?

I'm lying in the gutter, on the side of the road consumed by exhaust fumes. I don't want to die here, I thought. I can't. What was I even thinking of when I moved so far away from my family? What was I hoping to find? Have I already found it and I just don't know it? Is that why I am here now?

"Not again," my soul was crying.

"This can't be."

"I hadn't eaten anything for hours."

The taste of metal was like a leech sucking the moisture from my lips. Calcium had robbed my muscles of magnesium. My body was in turmoil, yet I felt calm within. The outer silver screen was action-packed with trauma. In contrast, slow peaceful music was playing in my inner space, the type that often sent me to sleep.

I was slowly drifting away. I knew it.

The fighter and the peacekeeper had reached a stalemate.

Drifting, falling, dropping—my connection with this reality was slowly dissolving. I was floating on a steady current into an abyss, on a conveyor belt heading to an unknown world, to a cloud frozen in time.

"This is it."

My life flashed before me in sensory intrusion.

"Mum, Dad, Paula, Mark…" my soul transmitted one last whisper in hope they would hear me.

"Nee, naw, nee, naw nee, naw…" Sirens could be heard in the distance. The sound was getting louder, closer. The traffic parted like two waves crashing in opposite directions, surrendering the center to create some flow. The ambulance had called my name.

"Please hurry," my soul cried. The other observers wished the same as the piercing sound got closer and even closer. How could peace exist when panic and noise were rife? Yet in this out-of-body state, there was silence and nothing was hidden. Invisibility had clarity. The onlookers couldn't hide any secrets. I could see beyond what I had seen before, watching the world with a panoramic aerial view from above.

The angels had given me wings.

Their lullaby fluttered through my heart.

"Let go!" they whispered.

"Fly."

I was tired of what seemed like a never-ending battle wherever I looked. I was working hard to forget my troubles, but I was spending all my earnings on temporary Band Aids or drugs to relieve the suffering of my life. Everything in my life leaned towards overprotection; I was always on high alert, fighting to survive in a world I did not truly understand. This had also extended to those who loved me. Despite my body crying out for some rest and reprieve, the primal survival mechanism kept it always on high alert, forever vigilant even as I slept. I was exhausted, desperate to break free from the shackles. The suffocating box was closing in on me. The hold had been too strong.

I was about to depart from this life, about to transform forever.

"We'll take over now," said the paramedics, arriving just in the nick of time, taking control of the situation.

I gasped for air.

Like a rubber band, my soul was snapped inward, back home. Its wings were instantly dissolved in the summer air. The angels' cries were replaced with sighs of relief. Chatter filled the air to disperse the bottleneck of nervous tension.

"Hold on," said my boyfriend, clasping my hand as I was placed into the ambulance. His touch instantly transported me back to the here and now. There is no time like the present. Actually, there is no time but the present. The present is the only time we have. We can't prove the past ever existed, and we are not certain if the future will ever come. His touch brought me straight to now, the power of now. Taking one moment at a time in the present would get me through this. I had returned.

The doors of the ambulance closed. When I opened my eyes again, it was to a profoundly altered reality.

As usual I was sent home from the hospital after a few hours of observation. There was no follow-up professional help, except instructions to take *prednisone*, used in the treatment of inflammation.

A week passed. Then I returned to the pub to thank the small group who had saved my life that day. I held my breath as I neared the local pub. My face flushed red as I crossed over the threshold. Embarrassment broke loose in my blood vessels like an infection, not because I had an allergic reaction in front of everyone the week before but because they had seen the spandex in all its glory. My sense of dignity, among other things had been shot to pieces that day. Of all the underwear to be caught in, it had to be the almighty spandex—especially in front of people I barely knew. These were people I had been trying to impress. People I knew I'd see again. So much for leaving a memorable impression—I'm sure this particular memory would be hard for them to forget. Coming back from a reaction was always like coming back to an apartment that had been rifled by thieves, with broken things all about. I had a sense of trying to pick up the pieces.

I thought of my mum for strength. And out of the blue, a surprise had come from Mum with her love. I'd been surprised when my boyfriend had told me there was a package for me to pick up at the post office. It wasn't close to my birthday. Christmas was months away. I hadn't ordered anything. Yet upon hearing what had happened, Mum had sent me the latest range of tartan-printed underwear on show in Ireland's high fashion stores. Bless her!

I generally never told my parents when I had an allergic incident. What good would it do to tell them the awful details when I was unreachable on the other side of the world? Nothing! It would only instigate more worry, stress, and pain and place them in a deeper state of helplessness. For some reason, though, I told mum about this incident. Maybe it was because her advice was: "Always wear clean underwear in case you get in an accident", and this motherly wisdom had instantly taken on significance for me. It made me laugh, but from that moment onward I swore to be mindful of my booty attire at all times. That gave me the strength to go forward.

Five years had now passed since I arrived in Sydney—my anniversary was literally upon me. By now I was single again, and I had moved to a nice beachside part of town, about a ten minute drive to Bondi. I had established a nice circle of friends and a wee humble abode where I could comfortably entertain and rest my head at night.

Mardi Gras time had come around again, and the city was all talk about the annual Gay and Lesbian Parade that passed down Oxford Street—the costumes, the excitement, the color of a night filled with partying and merriment. There was also Bondi beach the next morning for the revelers. But I wasn't interested in this. I had seen all this before. This year I wanted to have my own celebration—five years was a special milestone for me.

"We'll cook dinner for you this year," suggested my then flatmate, Sheila, while working out the anniversary celebration with two other friends, Tim and Nick.

"Ah! You know how I don't like that idea," was my reply, trying to persuade them just to have some drinks. They had heard about my allergies, but they had never seen the beast strike its intense blow.

"We can cook at my place," suggested Nick, offering the opportunity to eat out yet in a nice home setting. Little did I know but my friendship with Nick would evolve into a kinky weirdness by sun up.

Internal pressure to say "Yes" was bubbling just under the surface. My aim was to please, so to keep the peace, I gave in.

But this time there would be conditions.

"Let's all go to the supermarket together. Then I can check all the labels at the same time," I replied. "You can then cook using the food that I've approved." I was satisfied that this solution was a great idea. How wrong was I to think this!

"Michelle, what about this jar?" asked Tim, standing in aisle three, handing me a jar of pre-made sauce to get my seal of approval.

"No, that's not suitable. Sorry," I replied.

"Look here," I said pointing to the warning "This may contain traces of..." printed on the bottom of the ingredients' label.

"If it says 'this may contain' I can't afford to take any chances," I explained. "Trace elements are all it takes."

How can they possibly expect to decipher hidden ingredients when they don't yet know the basic ones? I thought, happy to have suggested this indirect lesson.

I can still recall feeling disgusted and upset a year later when this type of 'blanket' labeling of "may contain" had become more mainstream. Biscuits and ice cream had been instantly wiped off my diet, obviously not by choice but because the manufacturers feared litigation—putting a blanket screen on all their products with the words "may contain". It didn't matter if trace elements of peanuts or shellfish were present or not—the label could have listed arsenic as far as I was concerned. There was no way in the world I would go near these products ever again as long as the mysterious "may contain" raised the possibility of a red flag.

"Guys, honestly I am really happy to cook—seriously, I don't mind," was my final plea at the checkout to get them to change their minds. It didn't work.

I was feeling more than a bit antsy about this whole eating at Nick's place. But my friends were dead set on the idea to treat me—to put out the red carpet for me for a change. I always cooked for others. But I genuinely didn't mind. Cooking was something I really enjoyed. The hassle of entertaining was a small price to pay for the closest I'd ever get to sharing a meal with those I cared about. My mum had suggested that I take cooking classes when I was in high school. Mums always know best! I had learned to cook everything from scratch, as well as learned about food and nutrition, proving to be a key to survival when my allergic condition became more sensitive.

The four of us left the supermarket. We bought our liquor and beer and headed to Nick's place a couple of blocks away. I did one more final label check before Sheila and I retired into the living room. We listened to music while the boys cooked.

It was heaven.

"This is the perfect anniversary," I thought, but this thought was premature. It was in direct contradiction to what fate had in store.

The aroma from the kitchen was mesmerizing. Tonight the menu read chicken and vegetables. Even though the dish was a bit plain, it didn't matter. I was to eat among friends—the same meal as them, one that I hadn't cooked myself. I felt at ease. I had been involved in the buying process. I had read the labels, and everything had been wiped down before cooking commenced.

We joked, we laughed, we ate.

Then, I needed to go to the bathroom.

"Oh! No!" I tried to convince myself that I was imagining the all too familiar and unwelcome symptoms. This time my legs were on fire—they were itching like crazy—it was as if someone had thrown red burning fiberglass down my white trousers. The itch was spreading upward. The flight/flight response had kicked in. I didn't need this discomfort, aggravated by the heat of the last month of the Australian summer. I needed a shower. Cold! Something soothing on this flaring skin! I didn't suspect the allergen as the culprit; self-diagnosis convinced me that maybe I had developed a heat rash. I wasn't yet used to the hotter climate.

I turned to Nick.

"Do you have a pair of shorts I can borrow?" I asked, wanting to give my legs some air, not wanting to parade around in a G-string. He wandered off for a moment, returning with a pale blue striped pair of cotton boxer shorts.

"They will do, thank you," I said as I headed back to the bathroom. It felt weird trying on someone else's underwear, not to mention the difference in gender.

"Michelle," Tim called out.

No sound could be heard from the bathroom, except for the shower dripping. There was an uncomfortable pause as my friends waited for a signal.

"Are you okay?"

Again no answer! Eventually, they forced the door open to find out why. My body was slumped over the toilet; my white trousers had been replaced by red raw skin. The pale blue boxer shorts blended with my face. I had passed out.

"I'll call an ambulance," cried Sheila.

"We need to give her an injection."

Sheila remembered the training I had given her, just in case. She was my flatmate, and even though I had preferred to live on my own when single, we had become good friends. She had only moved in a couple of weeks before, so the allergy management training was still fresh in her mind. She rummaged around my purple barrel-shaped handbag with black feather trimming. I always carried a bag big enough to carry my EpiPen® (adrenaline auto-injector), the type with a shoulder strap, that to many appeared to be permanently fixed around my torso.

"Here, take this; I can't do it." Sheila's performance anxiety had set in, removing the safety cap and passing the medical device to the boys. I guess by now we had been drinking alcohol for a few hours and she didn't trust herself under the influence. Normally, I self-administered the auto-injector but I was unconscious.

I came to in Nick's bedroom, desperately gasping for air. Nick was holding my hand. Cries of panic could be heard outside the bedroom door, but inside it was calm. Nick kept his composure as we worked together to keep the peace while we waited.

I can best describe this as an altered state that occurs in the midst of an extreme allergic reaction. For me, everything felt numb, and there was no fear or pain. But despite the situation being borderline desperate, I can remember saying to myself, "Hold on." "Wait a bit longer." The initial fear dissolved, replaced with an overwhelming sense of peace and clarity. Somehow I knew and accepted that this peace was the action of my body in its attempt to use all of its resources to get through it. I knew that the first aid emergency protocol had been followed: take the adrenaline, call an ambulance, and try to stay as calm as possible.

At some point, we are all faced with life's traumas, and what we do when that happens is the great question. There is no set formula to predict whether a person will be broken or positively transformed by the event. I just knew it was all over if I let panic take control.

"There is more trauma on the other side of this door than in here," said the paramedic when he entered the bedroom. By this time, Sheila was crying uncontrollably in the living room. The whole contents of my handbag had been scattered all over the apartment amidst the panic to find the EpiPen®. The paramedic assisted me with my shoes. We made our departure for the hospital, which was only about a ten minute walk down the road. My friends would follow me later.

"We are so sorry," was the message from the boys when Sheila arrived. Only one visitor at a time was permitted in the emergency room. Incidentally, I would learn that a pre-prepared manufactured sauce had been added to the meal at the last minute. The boys felt that their culinary efforts had produced something bland, even tasteless. They checked the food label on the jar for nuts before they added its contents. They didn't think for one moment that there was any risk. To an untrained eye, the food appeared to be safe. They didn't know that hidden deadly codes existed. Why manufacturers use codes and numbers instead of stating the obvious always baffled me. You had to be an expert decipherer, as I was, to understand.

Sheila stayed with me for a brief moment. The emergency room was extra busy with Mardi Gras in full swing. It was 4 in the morning. Sheila soon departed, giving me $10 to pay for a taxi back to Nick's place, my mobile phone, and instructions to call her when I was discharged.

The emergency room doors slid open. The early morning sunlight blinded my eyes.

"Ring, ring, ring," there was no answer.

"Ring, ring…" it was 8 a.m., when most of the city was in recovery, slumbering after a big night.

"Ring, ring, ring…," there was still no answer.

"Come on, Sheila, pick up the phone," I said, jigging up and down in anticipation. "You have to answer." I didn't have any house keys to go home. She needed to let me back in to Nick's place. Also, $10 wouldn't cover a trip to my place. And I couldn't possibly get a bus in my current attire—a pair of boxer shorts, a three quarter length black top with an exaggerated fluffy collar trim, all topped off with three inch heels. To be wearing '70s style platform shoes while wearing male underwear wasn't a good look. I knew that I would have easily blended in with the revelers this weekend, but I had been through enough. I just wanted to go home, to sleep.

"Hello," said Sheila, sounding groggy, when she finally picked up the phone.

"I am in a taxi now. What is the actual address?" I asked. I didn't know the actual address or Nick's apartment number.

"The boys are asleep," replied Sheila as she looked around the apartment for a piece of mail, anything that had the address.

I was stressing. The meter had already clocked $8.

Time was money.

I didn't know where I was going. I wouldn't have enough to pay for the fare. Thank God Sheila was awake. She wouldn't be the only godsend that morning. The taxi driver, hearing my distress leaned over and turned off the meter.

"It's okay," he said when I got off the phone. "Everybody needs a helping hand from time to time…and it sounds like you need one now." I wanted to jump up and down with gratitude, to kiss him. This man, sitting only inches away, had truly come from heaven.

My anxiety about the taxi fare dissolved, but it was soon replaced by another concern. As we pulled up to the apartment, Sheila appeared, frantically waving her hands about to direct us to stop further down the road. The street had been littered with nuts. Just after the ambulance left, Nick went through every cupboard in his house to seek and destroy every nut in the apartment. They were thrown out of his window, three stories down, to land on the sidewalk. His supportive instinct to help a damsel in distress had delayed his core reaction—anger—which he took out on the nuts. I felt awful. The street mirrored my life, it was a minefield. I had to take each step at a time with caution, to avoid destruction, to avoid death. For the first time I realized that trauma had not only infiltrated my being that night, it had also infected my friends. As it turned out, my relationship with my flatmate, Sheila, would never be the same again. I had only shown her what to do in an emergency. I had never taught her how to cope with the before, during, and after a trauma strike.

Following every allergic episode, an investigation into finding the probable cause always ensued. To my surprise, I would discover that the food manufacturer had added a base sauce from another product range to that particular batch. The other range contained peanuts. In this instance, even if my friends had known how to decipher the hidden deadly codes, it didn't matter. They had no way of knowing this new deadly addition.

The following Sunday, Sheila and I met friends for a few Sunday afternoon drinks, Tim and Nick among them.

"It's great to see you," Nick said, waiting to greet me at the door. "It's okay. I made sure I didn't eat any nuts today," we embraced with a hug. This embrace was special, I was holding on to someone who had saved my life. Our friendship bond had evolved to a higher level.

"Where is Tim?" I asked, remembering that he had been sitting at the table when I arrived.

"Maybe he is in the bathroom," a friend replied.

"No, he's over there," another said, pointing to a table hidden from view in the corner.

I walked over.

"Hi," I said, but his eyes looked downward. Something wasn't right. He didn't want to be near me. He didn't want to speak with me. I could sense his rejection. He had been a good friend, I felt pain. The traumatic incident had obviously taken its toll. Maybe he just needed a bit of time? I walked away. But this niggled on my mind.

Had he rejected me because of guilt? Helplessness? Or not wanting to deal with anything associated with trauma—maybe ending our friendship was his trade off for peace. I would never know. But what I did know for certain—one common thread always follows life's traumas. In the aftermath of a trauma, a crossroads resides—a point to put our life under the microscope. It is a chance to re-evaluate our situation and to change the trajectory of it. The invisible sign on one side points to a path of "destruction and turmoil"—the other path leads to "peace and harmony". It is a point when the unconscious is yelling at us to make decisions or choices about our lives.

My friendship with Tim had been demoted to just being acquaintances. It would become nothing more than a memory, just like Paul, who had showed up when he did to save my life. I had had a lifetime to get intimate with trauma; my friends hadn't. Nobody had prepared them for this, except to fight, reject, avoid, or to go numb. Each of my friends had reacted to trauma according to their own background and experience: Sheila froze; Nick took his anger and fight out on nuts once he believed he had the situation under control, and Tim ran by rejecting or avoiding anything to do with trauma or drama—this included me.

I understood that men often respond to threat with fight or flight, whereas women and children more often freeze or go into paralysis. Could the difference be because men and women are generally conditioned from childhood to respond to threat differently? I knew from my own experience that my mental and emotional states in the midst of a full-blown allergic reaction were learned; they had been conditioned over time, from experience. This state assisted my body to do what it had to under extreme stress; it helped with recovery, but more importantly, it saved my life. But for the inexperienced, the unprepared, trauma, if left unaddressed, can hide like a parasite that burrows out of sight but which can eat away at you from the inside out. It goes so deep you don't consciously know it exists or that it can cause physical pain and suffering without you knowing the cause.

Pain by itself is just pain, but when pain is coupled with the understanding that it serves a purpose, then it is suffering. I could endure the suffering because my body had a reason for it to exist. Reactivation of pain if left unchecked gradually manifests itself into trauma. My body had become a master at recognizing trauma, a master of pain, of rejection. Dealing with the aftermath of this event had been no different than waking up in the morning, but to my friends, the pain of first time had cut deep. The intensity lingered, leaving a mark, a fingerprint.

I was used to it all. I lived on high alert. I didn't eat junk, processed, or takeaway food. I couldn't trust it to be safe. I never went near recreational drugs for fear I'd have a fatal allergic reaction, not from the drug itself but from sharing or passing a joint around that may have been contaminated with unsuspected allergens. I literally read the ingredients on everything that came with a label: moisturizer, shampoo, soap, food and drinks, deodorant, pet food, toothpaste, anything I came in contact with. It didn't matter whether it would be ingested, inhaled or touched, contact was contact.

I realized that my defense system had no reason to be continually on high alert, to be fighting against itself. But it was, and it did. Something had given it cause to kill peace—to misconstrue something harmless, nuts, as an enemy. The unnecessary turbulence in my life had to be peeled back like the layers of an onion. I had to seek and destroy this death sentence that had been bestowed upon me. My friends' defection was just one more reminder that I had to find a way to bring back peace into my life.

I was like a blood-stained warrior standing in the aftermath, of constant battle, inured to it all yet robbed of peace. To bring back peace, some of the fighter's reasoning had to be dismantled—fragmented programming that only served to provoke rather than to heal or to generate harmony had to be reprogrammed. While my friends were unused to trauma, I was too used to it—and I had to learn how to live in peace.

22

The Fighter Versus The Peacekeeper
"An overactive immune system needs peace
rather than more strength to fight."
Journal Extract: Michelle Flanagan

Over the years I read many books on how to strengthen
the immune system so as to boost my body's natural
power to fight. Yet I realized that when every ounce of
being is used to fight, well-being hangs in the balance,
for life is fuelled by nervous energy, restlessness, and a
lack of peace that borders on crisis. For me it only took
a tiny stressor such as a bit of criticism or just a smidgen
of pressure to tip the scales into fight mode.

My life had become a coiled spring attached to an emotional
rollercoaster ride; it was unpredictable, uncertain and could unravel
uncontrollably at any time. Despite being exhausted, I soldiered on. I
had to. I had no other choice but to warrior into the unknown, to fight
an enemy that I could not see. The fight got me this far. Without
staying in fight mode, my chances of survival would surely diminish.

By now I had spent most of the afternoon in Centennial Park.
Following my great grandmother's advice to go to a place in nature by
the water, this VIP day had proved invaluable. In these familiar
settings, memories of the past were flowing. I couldn't believe my
thoughts were of turbulence rather than a reflection of the serenity of
the setting. I knew that to give the fighter a rest, I had to surrender to
the peace of this place. The Australian sun was high in the sky; solace
was found under my favorite old tree that rested next to the small
white bridge, which was a metaphor for connection. This bridge joined
the forest with the murky swampland and the vast green open space.

A man passed by me, we engaged in a brief conversation.

"Nice day," he said. This was my cue to respond. How I chose to
respond was important as this would determine how we interacted

with each other. A simple "Yes" would have been sufficient but I chose to engage in conversation.

"Are you a professional photographer or is it a hobby?" I asked curious as he happily clicked his camera.

"I'm taking photos for the conservation society," he said.

His focus was on preserving this beautiful place, on recording or imprinting moments of nature—precious moments of life. His stress-free, cheerful appearance spoke of contentment in his work.

His accent was a dead giveaway that he was not from this place. It rang a familiar tune to my ear, from the same part of the world as I—north. Our place of origin was similar as was our ancestry. I felt a sense of connection to this passing stranger.

Would I have felt the same if we hadn't shared words? I wondered.

He had come to this park for the day from the Blue Mountains, a picturesque mountain range about an hour or so's drive outside of Sydney. He spoke about the most spectacular place to visit there—"The Valley of the Water; you must go there," he said. He suggested that I go deep into the mountains to discover this most amazing place. "This place will offer you more than you ever imagined." I can still recall him saying that. Was there a sense of irony in this conversation, a message to go deep into the mountains to find the most amazing place? For a brief moment I watched him adore nature through his lenses before he carried on his way.

My body was at rest. I felt rejuvenated and relaxed. Turmoil and disruption had temporarily dispersed.

A plane passed overhead. The roar of its engines could be heard for miles. The park wasn't far from the airport, but this alien sound was so far from this natural, serene place. What was it like hundreds of years ago when this sound didn't exist? I wondered. The sound of a truck rumbled in the distance, traveling along the outskirts of the parkland. Did birds and other animals have to adapt to these sounds? Are they even aware of these alien sounds? I pondered. These manmade sounds were once foreign to the native fauna so many years ago. Just like the fight/fight response that serves us in these times. In prehistoric times fight (resist) manifested by aggression or combat, and flight (submit) was to flee or run from a predator or life-threatening situation. The threat was literally real, in your face, in a do or die situation. In modern times threat can come in the form of a poor diet, over or under consumption, noise pollution, chemicals or toxicity, work-related stress, social interaction—the list goes on. Instead of using a spear to kill the threat as was the preferred method of early man, our fight response may manifest as anger or in arguments. Our flight mechanism is manifested by more modern means of escape—substance abuse, withdrawal from society, denial, avoidance, or dependency on others.

I sat in peace.

The old tree imparted its wisdom to me; fresh air touched my soul. I could hear mumbled voices in the distance. Tension began to bubble.

"Please stop swaying between peace and turmoil—it's exhausting," I told myself. "I need to rest, not fight."

Other people were approaching.

"Do I engage in another conversation or not?" I thought as I rested my pen on top of my journal. I couldn't see these people yet. This time I chose not to engage—to ignore them as they passed.

"But what if they are here to do me harm? I am on my own," I thought as they passed on their way. With so many bad things reported in the newspapers, threats to my safety did cross my mind. My body had automatically switched from a peaceful state to one of tension in a matter of seconds. It was on alert, just in case these people posed a threat. They passed without incident; no harm done. The switch to relaxation was reactivated.

Would I have responded in the same way if I had just been stung by a bee? I wondered. Especially knowing that bee stings in the past had sent me into a life-threatening situation?

The people's presence would have come as a welcome sight, potential life-savers rather than threats. As it was, their presence produced in me uncertainty, distrust, and tension.

Over the years I had learned that with every physical experience or event, an internal structure is created. That is, for every action there is a reaction, or systematic activity in the brain and body's nervous system. I had become more sensitive to food, and balance in my bodily systems had obviously gone askew. Somewhere along the way, a deep groove in the neural pathways of the brain was hardwired to link survival and the immune system as one, becoming the preferred method to maintain balance. Therefore, the innate healing power that deciphers the course of action necessary to replenish was relinquished to a system designed to fight.

Drama and turmoil had become a normal part of my life. Serenity had become alien to me. If any one day didn't contain a piece of drama, it didn't feel right. Drama, whether it was my own doing or was created by someone else, gave me a reason to live. It gave me a reason to exist. What I didn't know at the time was that even after the fight/flight response is long over, a resistance reaction allows the body to continue fighting the stressors long after the effects of the alarm system have dwindled. Is that why I was continually fighting? My body had never been given the chance to recover from intensity—to follow the angel's whisper—to let go.

With a history of avoiding conflict and an evident internal battle going on, could this also mean that I unintentionally avoided deeper parts of me? Conflict was within, so too was the essence of my authentic self—the bright shining diamond I was born to be. I had come to ignore, to avoid, to judge, to pass sentence on a crucial part of self. I had wiped it from my memory as unrelated. I had disconnected me from myself.

I had been caught in a vicious cycle, first set in motion by survival, but enduring as impairment. When the state of emergency or trauma is unresolved over long periods of time, the body reserves become depleted and the immune system weakens. Over nine years had passed since my arrival to Sydney. Every day had been a fight to stay alive. Now my immune system was attacking my thyroid gland as if a part of my own body was an enemy. If I wasn't willing to fight externally, the fight had obviously journeyed inward. Reflecting on the everyday conflict and struggle in my life, a mirror copy of this apparently now existed internally. There was an uncanny similarity to when my body waged an assault against a rich source of protein and healthy food— the peanut. Soldiers programmed to fight this so-called invader lay dormant in the darkness, just waiting for the right conditions to launch an assault, with me as the battleground.

A group of old people passed—they were slow on their feet, yet they were fit and jovial, evidently affected by the surrounding beauty. Water! The sound of water interrupted. My thoughts whizzed straight back to birth, to the life and survival a fountain of water brings to the body. Memories of sitting by the river as a teenager in Ireland intercepted.. Thoughts of the special place close to the crossroads where many tears had been spilled—tears that would eventually flow back into the river, one drop into the stream that gives life to something else. I sat and watched the stream for a while. It was never the same at any given time. This resonated with my life in so many ways.

"My body is a river—forever changing and moving," I thought.

"Are blocked or suppressed emotions just like rocks in a river?" I pondered. The river always finds a way to move around a rock blocking its path. Over time algae and grit remain, yet the river continually looks and finds a way to flow—the law of movement— energy in motion, e-motion. It only stops when a great wall or dam is created, or when drought or lack kills its flow.

After a lifetime of battles and limitations, the diagnosis of an internal war brought conflict home. I desperately needed some calm in my life. There had been too many rocks blocking my path. I wished that the constant worry, pain, and plague of uncertainty would somehow disappear. My body had been working on overtime, as if running at one hundred miles an hour to protect me, stretched to the limit as war was waged between parts of my body that were supposed to be friends.

My initial thought when diagnosed with the Graves Disease was to somehow work towards strengthening my immune system. But I realized that to give this system more power to combat an autoimmune-type disorder would also give it more strength to fight against my own body. Strength would only reinforce the stronghold in my fortress, the outer protective shell that had been created over time, which would rise to prevent the destructive nature of this new disease festering within.

In reality, this would surely create more internal conflict and possibly strengthen the urge to avoid, to run away, to ignore, to trance out. The body's dis-eased state would then never surrender or release its might so that I could have peace. It was as if my internal guide book on bodily and mental functions had been tampered with; as if some underlying force had taken control and erased some of the vital information my body needed to run efficiently. I came to realize that the allergen wasn't the problem; it was how my body was reacting to it that was. It wasn't any wonder that no "wonder" drug had been found to date to fix my allergies when something much greater had led to its existence and was keeping it alive. But what?

My defense system had taken over—my body was ruled by the system nature had intended to wage war, not peace. If I was to give a score, I'd say that protection was winning at 90% and healing at 10%. The immune system protects and defends the body from perceived threats to survival. It does not heal or replenish it. It creates blocks, to block potential invaders rather than to create flow. Its army of white blood cells is designed to fight, seek out, ingest, and kill invaders. Most of its soldiers hone in on a particular signal, a frequency transmitted by specific bacteria, fungal spores, viruses, etcetera. Like terminators they are programmed to seek out and destroy rather than to restore.

Some work tirelessly on the front lines, the high risk sectors known for threats such as bacteria and parasite infestation in the gut, fungal spores in the lungs, and so on. Without programming—a reason, or memory—these soldiers serve no purpose. They self-destruct; they do not see the obvious; they ignore. What if the region where these soldiers resided changed its unique frequency fingerprint? What if the flow or rhythm changed? Could this confuse their programming? Or even attract soldiers or foreigners from a different region that shared this new frequency? There had to be another system in place that could initiate action to keep the peace, to restore balance, to replenish, and to heal. That was the system I needed to find and strengthen.

If this healing system did exist, then I could assume that my immune system had waged war against it, or was protecting it. I hadn't changed my diet, as it was always under scrutiny. Was there something I had missed?

My immune system had become a dictatorship, using heightened stress and fear to dominate, to exploit the basic need for survival, leaving the healing system bound and gagged and only able to perform minimal tasks. This might explain why some parts of my body were showing signs of weakness: fear and anxiety were rampant, relaxation was stunted, my attention span was short, and my lack of conscious control meant that I could fly off the handle at even the smallest amount of stress. This was detrimental. We were not living in the world of the sudden attack of physical dangers, like saber tooth tigers. There was no need to live constantly on edge.

Why and how could I change this?

The many books I had read about survivors of cancer and other life-threatening health challenges spoke about an innate healing system in every cell of our bodies, a higher intelligence responsible for repairing damaged cells or tissue from an injury or illness and restoring the body back to a natural state of health. My cells regenerated all the time. The fact that they passed their learning onto the new cells was inspiring to me. My path of unfoldment indicated that memory could be altered, that it was dependent on the conditions of its environment. If I could alter the learning being passed to new cells, I could change my health. Just to think that a few million new cells were created just while reading the last two paragraphs in my journal blew my mind.

My body always knew when there was a threat; my defense system ran on a higher intelligence than I consciously did. The peanut butter contamination in the workplace; the boys adding pre-made contaminated food to my anniversary dinner; satay sauce in Washington; a kiss in Munich—the long list of the times my body's inner wisdom reacted was mind blowing. This revelation ignited a whole new set of questions.

Could I have been exposed to something else that had given rise to this 24/7 state of fight? Something my body was aware of but I counsciously wasn't? This was highly likely and probably why my immune system was constantly on high alert.

Was this system protecting me from something else? Was this why it couldn't rest? Why it had weakened over time, become more sensitive to the point where it had gone off the rails, protecting me from traces of utterly harmless substances? I needed to find out if there was anything else agravating my body that I was unaware of. I had been constantly vigilent for risky allergens, but I had never looked beyond that. The internal fighter was yelling "Charge!" for some reason, and I needed to find a way to calm it down.

But first I had to find out what all its fighting was about. In theory, if I discovered and removed other things from my life that my immune system had been stressing about, then surely it would give my body a break to reset itself, creating some time for it to heal.

But I faced another problem.

Except for my VIP allocated time, any remaining time was exhausted between my new job, doctors' appointments, and frequent blood tests. I couldn't spare adding the lengthy food elimination diets or skin prick tests onto my list, methods used in modern medicine to determine allergies.

I turned to the web to find an answer. Through relentless searching I would discover "hair testing." All I had to do was to send a sample of my hair in the mail, and within a few weeks I'd receive a report listing which foods and household products were compatible with my body. In other words, this list of foods and products would tell me what I COULD use to help repair my immune system, to calm the fighter down. Its focus was on restoration rather than on determining what I was allergic to.

What if the fighter's programming changed? It would surely have no reason to fight, to exist even. I instinctively knew that somewhere within the 'coulds' lay an answer. I was so impressed by this painless yet informative method of discovery, I would become a hair analysis consultant later. I still practise today. I do not tell you this to sell the hair analysis testing to you, but to let you know that I get an analysis done every six months so as to keep an eye on the fighter's activity. Armed with a list of over four hundred foods, metals, and household products, I am in a better position to pacify the fighter and keep it from fighting any unnecessary battles.

To my surprise, a particular brand of toothpaste showed up on my list of aggravators. It had been the only brand I had used since childhood. This is what really marked my journey into looking at other hidden ingredients such as fluoride, not only used in toothpaste but also used to cleanse the water I drank on a regular basis. By helping to calm the fighter, I could then turn my focus on the inner healer to repair and restore any damage. This leg of exploration would take me into the human nervous system. I would find out how, like a switchboard, our bodies continually switch between the fighter and the peacekeeper throughout every day. I also found that sometimes life can stick on one branch, thus causing detrimental damage. It can cross wires and create confusion between the senses.

Is the healing system the same as the defense system except with a different focus? It is undetectable by x-ray, but it is evidenced by its actions. When we cut ourselves, new skin is formed where the old layer was severed. Our body knits together a bone when it is fractured, tells us to eat when the stomach is empty, and regenerates and repairs damage to cells. A slower-acting system of the subconscious sends messages through physical symptoms, thoughts, emotions or dreams to warn of an imbalance in the body, or when we are in danger of losing health. I knew that to find resolution, I would have to look to some place deeper—to find the peacekeeper within that could talk some sense into the fighter. One thing I knew for certain: the body always knows that which the conscious does not.

I had become living proof that trauma if left unchecked can reinforce a "disconnect" between mind and body; it can fester as something incomplete, change conditions in the internal environment, and can be transferred from parent to child or generation to generation simply by mirroring the energetic blueprint. It can also lead to a variety of ailments and damage on a cellular level. I came to realize that trauma is similar in nature to avoidance. It also has two sides—energy potential that can be the catalyst to bring about positive creative change, or it can lead us on a path of self-destruction. A self-destructive path means that the fighter is winning.

It surprised me that post traumatic stress was never acknowledged as part of my recovery following every life-threatening allergic incident, especially when allergic episodes can strike at anytime. It was no wonder the fighter was in control when it already had a lifetime of unresolved destructive trauma on its hands, and why it couldn't rest even if it wanted to. I realized the importance of being aware that trauma has two-fold energy potential; to have the *courage* to embrace the unresolved repressed pain; to *forgive* the meaning behind it; and to move to the future by introducing more choices—to *let go*.

I was excited. I wanted to explore this healing system further. I turned to my basic needs for survival: food, water, air, shelter and reproduction as these were where I believed I'd find the hidden factor.

23

Insight Just under the Covers

"Every action carried out even when you sleep
can tell a lot about what you don't yet know.
Most healing happens when you sleep."

Journal Extract: Michelle Flanagan

Some misconceive sleep as simply "turning off" for a few hours and then "turning back on" upon waking. But I knew that whenever I got the flu, drifting off to sleep always seemed to help me recover somehow. Many scientific studies have reported that sleep deprivation can adversely affect the immune system. This tells me that there is a link between the immune system and sleep. But what else could it tell me?

My childhood aspirations to go to Art College came true when I left high school, a dream set since I was about two years old. I believe this path was written in stone long before I could talk. Was I just being primed with invaluable knowledge for what was to come later? Lessons such as the psychology of sleep, dream symbols and their meanings, then passed off as irrelevant or only specific to creativity would resurface on my path of healing. I would realize that there was more to sleep than I had imagined. Dreams not only access creativity and imagination, but they are also a direct link to what is going on within— they are the open door to the unconscious.

Memories may not be present in the conscious mind, but no information or experience is ever lost. Absolutely all information, including imagination and creativity, are stored in our unconscious. This knowledge and more would filter its way back into my consciousness almost twenty years later. Only three months into my foundation year, the college had successfully immersed me into the world of imagination beyond consciousness—they would teach me how to listen to my dreams and to decipher their codes. My lecturers recognized that learning to analyze dreams was an open door to creativity, imagination, and ultimately to the subconscious mind. But for me, just like learning to decipher what codes on food labels meant, I loved deciphering if there was more behind my dreams.

We were asked to record our dreams, to set our alarm clocks every morning to wake up a couple of hours before our usual waking time. Every morning when I was still a bit groggy, I was to write down what I had dreamt about in a notebook. The key was to make sure that I recorded as many details as possible, as a detail might clarify a particular situation, deliver a message, and/or deliver an insight. But I normally fell into a deep sleep and only recalled dreams here and there. Over time it surprised me that just intending to remember before I fell asleep was enough to train myself to remember—the recalling of dreams began to flow.

My teacher told us that dreams usually occur in a series as different aspects of a specific complexity. She said that over a period of time such as a month, all the pieces illuminate to reveal different perspectives or an all-rounded picture of the overall complex. The same applied to the physical unconscious body. Over time I had learned to recognize that sleep is when the body and mind process all the data accumulated through daily experiences, when it digests food, thoughts and emotions, heals damages, replenishes, and regenerates cells. That said, my sleeping patterns always stuck out as unusual for as long as I could remember.

Even though it often took me a while to fall asleep, when I did it was deep, deep, deep, as if I had been teleported out of this world—maybe I had, but how could I know? From childhood into my adult years, I'd sleep curled up at the end of the bed, hoarding all the covers. Unbeknownst to me, I slept on the side of the bed closest to the exit, and others often joked about the hop, skip, and jump I made every morning, as if on hot coals, from the bed to the door. It was comical. If woken unexpectedly from a deep sleep in the early hours of the morning, I was enraged—fuelled by high charges of energy surging through my body. I was often confused as to where all this energy had come from, especially when my body was supposed to have been in a restful state. I'm sure I scarred my mum with flying shoes projected in her direction—a common occurrence when she woke me every morning for school.

But I will never forget waking up every morning to the first and only thought flashing through my mind being that of survival: "Will I make it through the day?" My mind was preparing itself for the day-to-day adaptation that lay ahead. Any early morning pressure to rise and shine gnawed at my soul—I needed time to start a new day.

Sometimes, when under extreme stress, I'd wake in a cold sweat. Nightmarish images of crocodiles were just another recurrence of a dream that had haunted me for as long as I could remember. Although my mum could tell me that problems at bedtime had arisen when I encountered the ear problems that plagued me since I was a child, this recurring dream baffled me.

I had learned that it is normal for a healthy toddler to occasionally fear the dark and monsters, especially around twenty months when exploration of imagination and fantasy takes on a new meaning. The young mind is unable to tell the difference between fantasy and reality. Basically I believed everything I saw on television back then was real. I can still recall my sister teasing me at Christmas. I was about five years old at the time, and she had just turned seven. It was a time in my life when Santa and the magic surrounding Christmas was very real. Nobody had told me anything different.

I can still hear the sleigh bells ringing. It was Christmas Eve, when anticipation fills the hearts and minds of the young around the globe waiting for Santa's arrival. Tucked in by Mum, I can still recall this night as being one of excitement rather than fear. The smell of cinnamon and pine infiltrated the air. We had just been bathed, my sister, brother and I, in preparation for Christmas day. I wore my favorite red pajamas, they smelled warm and fuzzy, and I swaddled in cleanliness from head to toe. Santa would be good to me this year, I just knew it. He couldn't miss me this year even if he tried. I was a bright shining radiance, squeaky clean inside out.

"Do you hear the bells?" my sister asked. By now Mum had retired back downstairs to the living room. The distant hum of the television in the living room could be heard. Ignoring this, my ears were trying to hone in on Santa's signal, the sound of his sleigh bells, the evidence of his arrival. Maybe this is the year, I thought, trying as hard as I could to stay awake in hope that I'd be lucky this time to catch a glimpse.

"Listen, Michelle," she repeated. "Can you hear the sleigh bells?"

I jumped out of bed, pulling back the curtains, and the starry night unfolded before my eyes. Icicles glistened on the window sill as I pressed my nose up against the cold darkness. I watched, moving my eyes from right to left. My imagination hadn't kicked in yet. All other sounds apart from what I wanted to hear had been blacked out. This brought disappointment—unfulfilled expectations—nothing. Santa was nowhere to be seen.

"Look over there," Paula said, pointing to a tiny spot in the distance. Far beyond the neighborhood buildings, a slight glow of red could be seen.

"Yes, I see it," I said, growing excited. But I had seen this light many times before. But tonight its prior existence was ignored. I really wanted to believe that it was Santa's favorite reindeer. Stories had told that Rudolf's bright red nose guided the way. I believed them.

"Jingle, jingle, jingle." the faint sound of bells suddenly entered my ears. "I can hear it!" I was now a believer. My body couldn't contain the excitement as I danced around on my bed. He was close. This would be my year to meet Santa. I couldn't wait to tell my friends at school. Hope increased as the sound got louder, as too the tiny dot in the distance grew bigger and closer. I could finally see this guide in full view, as clear as the brightest star.

"There he is," I said, glowing, even though urged by my sister to rest my head on the pillow. "Santa can't see that you are awake," she said in an ever so matter of fact way. This familiar rule of Christmas squashed my plans.

My ear rested on the soft, freshly scented cotton pillow.

It smelled of home, of comfort, of safety.

I lay waiting with eyes closed. I listened as the jingle dissolved into the recesses of my imagination. Again, anticipation had turned into nothing.

"He's not coming, is he?" I asked.

Reality had taken a bite.

"Ha! Ha! I fooled you," said Paula.

"He was never there in the first place," she admitted, telling me that the sound came from the television downstairs. I gently bit my quivering lip as this dream rapidly faded into the darkness, shattered like stardust lost in the galaxy of wishes washing over the night sky.

"I really did see him," I thought, trying to convince myself of this existence, desperate to hang onto hope. It was hope that kept me going. But life lessons would later teach me that hope also closed my mind from venturing outside the precious ring of hope I had created, tying me to something I couldn't prove ever existed—the past. Reality and fantasy were all but one. They had no difference. Santa was well and truly real in my childhood eyes. No matter how hard I tried to stay awake, my eyes got heavy and I drifted off to sleep.

Somehow this particular memory had found its way back to me over three decades later. This surprised me. Like too many other memories I had once forgotten, these memories as opposed to others had bubbled to the surface as soon as I began to look for specifics and ways to express feelings and thoughts bottled within.

As soon as I remembered this story, I remember laughing to myself. This had been a typical childhood experience, yet by it resurfacing, I knew that something about it had been left unresolved. As soon as it came to the surface, the unresolved without much conscious thought was released forever, reclassified as a wonderful childhood moment— as seen through the eyes of an adult.

I retrieved my dream notebooks kept in my old bedroom in Ireland since 1989, and through recording my dreams again, I set out to explore the connection my subconscious mind had with crocodiles. To my surprise while reading my notebooks again, two entries written in 1988 stood out—one that I was in Australia, living by the beach, sitting in the afternoon sun; the other that I was at a feast in heaven eating absolutely everything without the fear of an allergic reaction. This made me realize that there was more to dreams than I had initially thought.

I wondered why I had stopped recording my dreams when they told me so much, making a vow to start recording dreams from that moment onward. I was curious to discover what else had I stored in my mind. To my surprise, it didn't take long before an early memory that had been long forgotten bubbled to the surface.

"It's okay; the crocodiles are hiding; we can make a run for it," Paula said, coaxing me to take one more step over the threshold. Again I was about five years old. Just like Santa's bells, these words would ring an unconscious faint hum in my head and body for another thirty-two years. Although we were only sixteen months apart, my elder sister's words echoed in my young innocent ears. Hearing from her that crocodiles lived in the dark spaces under my bed was very real.

"But we have to hurry, because they will eat you," she said. Tasting fear through remnants of toothpaste on my lips while clutching my flashlight firmly as the weapon of choice, I made preparation to hop, skip, and jump on top of Paula's bed to mine. The key was to avoid setting foot on the bedroom floor.

"Girls, have you brushed your teeth?" my mum called out, hearing our chatter on the landing at the top of the stairs. "I'm on my way now to tuck you in," she said. We heard her footsteps getting closer.

"Quick, we better go now, because Mum won't be happy if we are not in bed," my sister said, initiating the nightly balancing act in flight across the room, landing to the sound of crackles from the plastic sheet as protection from wetting the bed. Bed-wetting was a great cause of distress at that age.

Every night I followed the same routine, encasing myself in the covers, my security blanket as protection from the crocodiles. I slept at the end of the bed, believing this to be the perfect position to fend off any danger. Unknown to me, elements of this behavior had carried into adulthood.

While recollecting this dream for about the hundredth time, if I was to describe this nightmare, it might go something like this:

"I feel safe in my slumber, wrapped in a womb-like cocoon, the soft fluffy quilt of warmth, indifferent to the outside world. My mind is at rest, and my body relaxed, calm, and quiet, with my eyes closed to any outside disturbance by the constant bombardment on my senses when I am awake. I drift deeper. It's my own private viewing of the movies within, breathing is slow and at a steady pace, drifting even deeper into this dream state.

Slow brain waves stir the cavalry of restorers who reside in the space between the spaces. Their overall mission is to scan the territory for imbalance or unrest, to maintain balance and restore order between other squads or systems. Each has his own mission which is to protect, to fight, to digest, to build, to repair, to eliminate, to regulate, to remember, to beat, to decipher, to breathe.

The restorer liaises between organs, tissues, and cells; it fine-tunes and manages the demands of constant shifts and changes, fixes damages, and ultimately keeps the peace.

My eyes, like butterfly wings, begin to flutter rapidly as the restorers move through each area: scanning, evaluating, and sending data to the great information database for processing. The movie has begun. Salivation increases, moisture dribbles on the pillow, this indicating the hive of activity now taking place in digestion. Digesters and eliminators are hard at work. This is the only moment they can really get their jobs done. Each to her own, they have come to the digestive system to perform particular tasks. Bile salts found in the liver/gallbladder are busily absorbing fat in the intestines, the pancreas has sent digestive enzymes to digest food eaten earlier, to break down starch, fat, and protein, and to extract energy and nutrients for fuel.

The restorer pays particular attention to this area, because food lists as one of the basic necessities for survival. Any imbalance, parasite, or harmful bacteria present that can prevent this system from doing its job properly could lead to starvation. It goes through its basic survival checklist for that area: water, air, food, shelter (environment), light, and reproduction (cells).

In this instance an imbalance is noted. Stage 2 is initiated to mediate between other bodily parts in an attempt to restore balance. If air is needed, a signal is sent to the brain telling it to take a breath. If posture inhibits blood flow, a signal is sent instructing me to move in the bed. In this instance, the environment is too acidic, and other problems emerge. The kidneys that govern water metabolism have weakened over time by over activity of the adrenal glands on top, aggravated by a constant influx of displaced energy. The restorer recognizes that a build-up of fear encapsulated from that day has raised acid levels. But calcium is depleted; it is normally absorbed to restore Ph balance, and the part of the adrenal glands which regulates non life-threatening stress is overworked.

It calls on the commander of the glands, the pituitary, located at the base of the brain. One of its assignments is to balance water, but all reservoirs are low. Water, another vital necessity on the survival checklist, is in threat. Therefore, Stage 3 is initiated. An alert is sent through the nerves to the amygdala, a primitive part in the brain that has evolved since the origin of humans. It works faster than its thinking counterparts and is imperative for survival. With the help of the glands commander, the emergency response team in the other part of the adrenals is called to duty.

As my brain can't tell the difference between what is fantasy or real, images and sounds of my worst fears emerge, sending a shockwave of physiological shifts throughout my body. The restorer knows one of my greatest fears since childhood, and it sets out to recreate the scene on my internal movie screen.

I find myself drifting in swampland, caught in dark murky water, surrounded by crocodiles. I will be their next meal if I don't find a way out. My heart begins to race as they get closer. I need to get to the bridge, but my boat is stuck in the reeds. There's not enough water to release. I must release to survive.

My breathing rate increases, filling my lungs with air; inhalation and exhalation are shallow. Partly digested food now sits on pause. I'd be in a state of paralysis if it wasn't for the adrenaline now surging through my body. A warm and fuzzy dream of being surrounded by hugs intercepts—this an attempt by the restorers to secrete the cuddle hormone to reduce the stress hormones surging through the blood. The crocodiles are too strong and re-enter the scene.

The smell and taste of fear is now sucking my mouth dry through remnants of toothpaste. Sweat pours through every pore in my skin, and goose bumps appear as capillaries constrict close to the surface of my skin. Hair rises on the back of my neck—the adrenals are active. My muscles tense, moving frantically as I grab a metal bar, ready to fight. I toss and turn in the bed. My sense of smell is stronger now as the threat gets closer. The biggest crocodile I've ever seen in my life is right beside me.

I can't move.

I'm stuck. My body is in paralysis.

Sheer terror is flowing through my veins.

My mind is only focused on one thing: that is to survive.

The crocodile lunges from the darkness, revealing its underbelly mid-flight. What do I do? I hold my breath and brace for impending doom. I know that it's only moments before impact. An earth-shuddering scream erupts from the build-up of air in my lungs. It wakes me up, momentarily stunned.

"Phew! It was only a dream."

I gradually come around to reality with a sense of relief. The sheets are damp with sweat, indicating that my body did actually experience something. I am confused.

Burning sensations linger in my kidneys telling me to go to the bathroom, but my mouth is dry, so I take a drink.

Somewhere along the way, this sequence of events in combination with the maturing of the central nervous system caused a mismatch of information, distortions linking the sequences of memories as one. It was only a matter of time before images of crocodiles would be linked with fear, a common feeling at bedtime. Gradually, as I got older, the original childhood memory was forgotten, but a phobic nervous response to crocodiles remained. It was a fear dialed up or intensified so much that the information somewhere in between was lost.

Eventually I became so terrified of crocodiles that even watching these reptiles on TV, hearing about them in conversation, or just thinking about them was enough to infuse highly charged shockwaves of fear through my body. I was primed to react, whether I was consciously aware of the underlying triggers or not. Forgotten sequences, lost memories that had fallen through the cracks, reappeared as clear as a summer's sky, when the right ingredients were present. Maybe this was because I revisited my dreams through intuitive writing.

When a build-up of fear reached a pinnacle in my body, I was prone to urinary tract infections (kidneys) and recurring nightmares of crocodiles. These are just two examples of how I believe the unconscious attempts to release and restore balance. The restorer, even though it works 24/7 behind the scenes, runs at its optimum during sleep, or when the body and mind are deeply relaxed and calm.

Now I was awake.

What of the brand of toothpaste I used in childhood? I wondered if every time I brushed my teeth with the same brand of toothpaste before going to bed as an adult, that I set up a precursor to how I slept, that it was an unconscious anchor linked to a childhood fear of crocodiles and feelings of intense anxiety just before falling asleep.

Dreams can sometimes allow us to experience an unresolved emotion our healing system wants to release or wants us to consciously notice. Dreams bubble up from the core of our being from innate wisdom itself. Our ancient ancestors understood this, believing that dreams came from a level beyond time and space from the spiritual world. Therefore, they treated them with the utmost respect. Dreams and the link to bodily functions fascinated me, therefore I began to delve even deeper into this area to see what I could find. The results would surprise me. I found that each organ of the body had its own dream story to tell.

Although I have only scratched the surface, dreams highlight just how much information we can find out about our unconscious body. In our dreams, unresolved problems are acted out, so it can be beneficial to learn or have someone decipher their meanings. Observing changes in sleeping patterns, recording dreams, and learning how to interpret them is an open door to the giant within——the unconscious mind, body, and soul. Once thoughts and feelings are expressed, the underlying problems begin to be resolved.

Up until now I had forgotten that the unconscious cannot tell a lie, even if the truth is suppressed. Few people listen to the open door to the unconscious—dreams. Dreams vary in importance from releasing the relatively unimportant stresses of the day early in sleep to the more significant and deep subconscious-seated dreams that occur later at night. Every cell in our body goes back to how we evolved as human beings. We are transferring energy from cell to cell on a daily basis. If the information or cell memory is anchored to a message from the past, the unconscious will hold onto it until we become aware of the message. Once the choice is made to take this message on board, only then can it be released.

Although I uncovered the link between my crocodile nightmare and intense fear, somehow I instinctively knew that there was more to this puzzle when it came to unraveling my path to healing.

What did I know about sleep? Only that it is something fish, animals, and humans must do, and therefore it has to be of great importance. I was curious to find out why bats sleep upside down, horses standing up, while killer whales and some dolphins do not sleep in their first month. Some animals hibernate for the winter, some sleep in packs or groups, some aquatics swim even though they are asleep, while others have one side of their brain awake. Koala bears, a native mammal of Australia, can sleep up to nineteen hours a day.

Studies have shown that hunter-gatherer and other nomadic tribes of the past survived by sleeping "on" and "off" throughout the night, sleeping in groups for warmth and protection from predators' eyes. They respected the rhythms of the night and day, were in tune with nature, and believed that dreams came from the spiritual world.

Archaeological evidence suggests that they were relatively healthy, that arthritis was uncommon, and the most frequent causes of death were due to trauma from predators, hunting, and other accidents related to primitive life conditions.

The hunter-gatherers that exist today, such as the !Kung of the Kalahari Desert, also survive by adapting to their surroundings. They sleep outside unless the weather is bad; they also sleep in groups with extended family. The spiritual world is in every part of their lives. They are known to dance around the fire in trance under the stars well into the night. Cancer, obesity, diabetes, asthma, allergies, hypertension, and heart disease are uncommon among these people. Survival appears to be the main driver behind their sleeping habits: external factors such as climate, protection from predators, seasons, habitat, food, and water. I was curious to explore what happens internally, and if there might be a link or a clue to my situation.

Nightmares—flashbacks of the rape in Munich were now transmitting at an all time high. Something had triggered this gun to go off. These occurrences didn't surprise me. I was within range of the two month anniversary window of this incident. The date was fast approaching, the cue to tell my tormentors to get closer in my dreams. This was the time when these ghosts were particularly hungry for repetition. This time scared me—a heightened chance of drifting into the arms of these demons. The thirteenth year since the initial incident was getting close. Sleep leveled its paralyzing blow, which buckets full of caffeine couldn't keep away. As if the incident had only happened yesterday, I was re-living my own Elm Street nightmare over and over again. I didn't seem to have any control over it. Even daydreams were interrupted by it.

I was afraid to fall asleep or drift off into my own world for fear my tormentors would catch me unaware as they did before—snatching my deepest essence in my sleep. I desperately needed some calm and relaxation in my life. I was growing weary, tired, and irritable. Tiredness ruled my life. I woke up tired. I worked through the day feeling tired. I rested my head on my pillow every night, exhausted. My mind played out a living torture day after day—sleep deprivation took hold. I couldn't wait one more day for this storm to pass, to the day after when the sun shone again, to when the tormentors released some of their grip for another year. Insomnia needed to be outlawed. And fast. I was desperate to explore every option.

This is when I took my first class on meditation. I just wanted to sleep—to relax. Not only did I learn about Solfeggio frequencies at this course, I would also learn about different levels of consciousness. Even though I didn't realize it at the time, this introduction to levels of consciousness would prove invaluable on my path of healing. I would explore how different brainwave frequencies determined whether I was awake, daydreaming or in a deep sleep; whether I had lots or thoughts or none at all; that specific brainwave frequencies dictated behavior, what I saw, heard, felt, craved, smelled, tasted, or didn't. And that these brainwaves could be retrained simply by making subtle changes in my day-to-day life.

I would come to the realization that my body had attached the date of the rape incident to the memory of it. Somehow this didn't surprise me. The trauma happened around an annual event—Munich literally transformed at a certain time every year—an event which is advertized almost everywhere. And every person who had been assigned to my mental health care most always asked for a date.

"When did the rape occur?" I can still recall the usual question—like clockwork, it was as if my body locked in at this time of the year to be on the alert. Do you remember what you were doing when "Princess Diana is dead" was announced over the wire? Or what you were doing when the horror of 9/11 unfolded? I do. And as each year passes since these particular events, what I was doing back then also resurfaces—the date, time of year, or media reminders are more than enough to trigger the memory of what I was doing or where I was in my life when these incidents occurred. This made me realize the grip time had on the rape incident and other traumatic events I had encountered in the past. This grip with time needed to be released. This was something I had to take into my own hands—only I had the key to release these ghosts of the past. My own personal exorcism was required, a cleansing to wake from this turmoil.

With my most vulnerable time being just before sleep, I believed that it was important to develop a method or routine to help me fall asleep at bedtime. Otherwise, unless cleared, festering fear and anxiety would linger and conflict when the restorer did most of its work while

I slept. I couldn't afford this on my path of healing. The restorer needed to work unimpeded.

Often, when I had trouble sleeping because of too many shopping list type thoughts flowing through my head, I began to create what I now call a "Universe To Do List". This is simply writing down on paper a "To Do" list prior to sleep of things that needed to be done in the near future. Three items are placed on the right hand side—things I know without a doubt I will achieve the following day: for example, wake up, get out of bed, and get dressed. On the left hand side, I create a "To Do" list for the UNIVERSE or my inner intelligence to take care of. The key is to TRUST without fail that the universe will accomplish this. When the universe's item is achieved, I award it with a sticker, normally a gold star to acknowledge and reward the effort. At first I was skeptical as to whether this would work or not. But, I was in desperate need to fall asleep without feeling terrorized, before, during, and after sleep.

Gradually over time, I noticed the more I created this list, the more I realized that I had an ally to assist with my wants and wishes. One example that springs to mind is when I started my new job in the city. I wanted to drive to work rather than take public transportation so that I could minimize the risk of coming into contact with allergens, but I didn't have a space to park my car, and city parking proved too expensive. I wrote on my Universe To Do list to "Find a cheap parking space".

To my surprise, the day after I wrote this, an email from a local city resident circulated around the office, offering to sublet her garage space for minimal weekly rent. As soon as I read the email, I knew without a doubt that this was the workings of the universe. I called the woman straight away and got the parking spot, while secretly thanking the universe for manifesting this.

Not only does this process create a sense of fun and intrigue, it also helps to clear feelings of being anxious or overwhelmed just before drifting off, thus enhancing the quality of sleep.

When first learning about meditation I found that it can retrain the nervous system such that if there is *sympathetic* nervous system dominance, meditation can switch the nervous system to the *parasympathetic* branch (Appendix: The Nervous System). But, despite knowing this, my mind was too active to sit still for any length of time.

I had to be busy. If I wasn't, I became bored very easily. When I was bored, I took risks. I'd squander what little money I had and paint the town red. I personally found meditation boring at the beginning despite it being a very effective method to adjust brainwaves. My interest lay in exploring body entrainment tools further.

Sitting listening to sound frequencies was more appealing to me. I had learned that the brain literally follows along with stimuli in proximity. For instance, if lights flash at a rate of four cycles a second or if a drum beats at the same rate, the brain will mimic the rate with its own brainwaves. The body automatically follows whatever the brainwave frequency is. For instance, we are normally asleep at four brainwave cycles per second—so if light was to pulsate at this rate, it can put a person to sleep. I also discovered that a red-colored light placed beside the bed automatically turned the *parasympathetic* branch of the nervous system "on", whereas a blue light (blue sky) activates the *sympathetic* branch. (See Appendix: The Nervous System)

I found this knowledge useful when I had trouble falling asleep. I would return to meditation later, once I had more of an understanding of the mind-body nature of a reaction. I needed to figure out what might regulate consciousness in the body, and fast— before any other illness materialized.

"What organ might do this?" I asked myself, searching through all my boxes of information collected over the years. I came across an article about sleep that mentioned the regulator of wake/sleep patterns and seasonal functions. The answer pointed to a small gland called the "pineal" located deep in the center of my head. Like an internal clock, it regulates the 24 hour cycle (circadian rhythms) of biochemical, physiological, and behavioral processes. Its actions are dictated by external cues in the environment, the primary one of which is daylight. But this doesn't only synchronize the body according to light and dark; other factors such as meal time, artificial light, exercise or lack thereof, stress, seasons, reminders such as anniversaries, internal environmental factors such as hormones and blood quality/flow, are all factors of influence.

Even organ function seemed to switch "higher" or "lower" during their set times throughout each day. Knowing this information would prove invaluable as it gave me some control over my day-to-day emotions and well-being. This told me an approximate time when to focus on a particular part of the body on my healing path. For instance, if I was particularly worried about something between 7-9 a.m., I'd acknowledge the feeling and revisit it later, knowing that my stomach (seat of worry) was most active at this time. This could explain why on occasion I woke up feeling particularly worried about one thing or another, triggered at this time. And if I woke between 1-3 a.m., I'd more than likely feel angrier than normal, or the dream I just had may have included a fight or hostile environment. I'd know that this was my inner healer at work, releasing the energy of anger (conflict) which I avoided during waking hours.

I hypothesized that if the pineal gland controls the various bio-rhythms of the body, then it must also be able to communicate with or "talk" to all the organs, the systems, even each individual cell. If indeed true then this might be the key to unlock the doorway to change unwanted reactions on a cellular level. Just thinking about this possibility excited me.

24
Communication on All Levels
"Look deeper and there you will find the master communicator within."
Journal Extract: Michelle Flanagan

Every time I had an acute allergic reaction, I'd receive a call from Dad a few hours later from the other side of the world just to make contact. He didn't know anything about the most recent incident except that a dream had alerted him to urgently call me.

"Michelle, I just had a very upsetting dream, and needed to call to check that you are okay," my dad's panic-stricken voice came through from the other end of the phone. Rather than worry or upset him any more than was necessary, I glossed over the last few hours of the traumatic experience, thus eliminating any more cause for panic or worry as the initial threat was over and I was in recovery.

In fact, the times I told my parents about the anaphylactic encounters were rare. Most life-threatening incidents were too painful for them to hear about. Being on the other side of the world only brought more helplessness to the forefront. What could they do? To avoid any suspicion of my cover up, from time to time an incident was leaked into their consciousness. One of these leaks that sprung to mind was when I got caught in spandex. It fit my personal disclosure criteria checklist; any trauma associated with the incident could be sidetracked, the horror could be easily replaced with humor.

But it always baffled me how they always knew regardless when something awful had happened.

"Dad, it was just a bad dream. Don't worry. I am fine," I said, to make the worry seem insignificant. I used every ounce of energy I had to sound uplifting, hiding the truth.

"I had an awful dream that peanuts took a hold of you, and I heard you crying for help," he continued as goose bumps appeared on my skin. "Please, always be careful," he said in a calmer voice, obviously reassured to hear that everything was fine.

He was in Ireland and nobody could have told him of the recent incident. I hung up the phone stunned, but would later learn that as my medical incidents became more frequent, so too did his very timely calls asking if I was okay.

How did he know? Did I have a built in transmitter broadcasting every traumatic experience I encountered and he was tuned into my frequency? These calls always stuck out as something odd; the timing was almost surreal. I wondered if there was more to them than met the eye, and if an inner intelligence had been trying to tell me something at the time. This unexplained phenomenon baffled me. It seemed to illustrate people's ability to communicate on a level beyond conscious comprehension.

Since the day I was born, communication has been a big part of my life. I grew up surrounded by my dad's passion for movies, cameras, television or anything else that could send or receive signals to communicate.

"Our family was one of the first on our street to have a color television." I can still recall dad proudly recalling the early years of my life. Unlike today, to have a color television back then was a MAJOR deal. Actually, even to have a television was big.

On rainy days—of which there were many in Ireland—I can still recall playing in Dad's mini movie theater; a shed located at the end of the garden of my first family home. Instead of fairies living at the back of the garden, fairy tales came to life on our own movie screen. He had converted the shed to house seating for a small group of about ten people, complete with a retractable screen at one end and a small box room located at the other. This served as a miniature version of the movie projection room one might see in a cinema. This box had just enough room for one person and a projector. Through a small window about the size of a standard book, Dad projected precious memories onto the screen. Family movies; winning my first gold medal for running at the local community games; singing at my first Holy Communion, even though the angel's lullaby had been left at home; birthday parties with friends at home; the aftermath of Santa's annual visit, showing off what he had bestowed on me: paints, paintbrushes, canvas, sketchbooks, and crafts; the first time I set foot on a plane, my first impressions of a foreign place caught on film; our family dog Kim, a light brown cocker spaniel; this special place projected a multitude of forgotten memories that had been captured in time. It was special, considering the world of television was only emerging.

I was probably one of the most filmed children in the world. Having access to these photos and memory snippets would prove invaluable on my path of healing later. All it took was an image, smell, sound, taste, or touch to instantly trigger a memory from the past, the transporters to a specific moment once forgotten—and once remembered, it was released into the air like a bird taking flight.

On days when the sun did decide to show its face, we children would play on our slide and our two swings, or muck around in a sand pit, or join hands as we sung "Ring a ring a rosy" while circling around a large pole, the centerpiece of the back garden.

I didn't really know what the pole was for except that it was a little taller than our house and gave Dad great joy when the picture on his television was crystal clear. My dad has always been ahead of his time when it comes to technology; so much so that he now owns two businesses: one that specializes in security alarm systems and the other in TV and DVD production and studio hire. I can understand the latter, but I had always been curious about how he got into the security business. Especially knowing that his father was a painter and decorator in his day—another creative type.

I can still remember the day I asked him why and found his answer quite unexpected yet rather amusing.

When my parents moved into their home as newlyweds a community problem had become evident. All the women in the area were experiencing an underwear shortage, especially of a sensual nature. Somehow, ladies' underclothing would mysteriously disappear from the clotheslines in the early hours of the morning. The neighborhood had a ladies' underwear bandit! This bemused the local police, who advised a twenty-four hour neighborhood watch in the hope that they would catch the apparent thief. Months passed, and the booty attire continued to go missing.

Dad decided some intervention was required, some creative thinking. He had a different plan. Instead of neighborhood watch, he got permission from the locals to run cables through each garden linking their clotheslines to a makeshift alarm. This came complete with lights and sensors to detect any movement. The next time the underwear bandit came out of the darkness, creative thinking would expose this booty caller. It worked; the bandit was caught. The plan was rather ingenious because not only did they catch the culprit, but this novel and unusual story hit the local newspaper. Dad had received an offer from a U.K. security company to head their business in Ireland. He accepted. Without realizing it, he had entered the alarm business.

I can still recall the day when we moved to our second family home on the outskirts of Dublin. For about a week Dad's face was distant, something had him preoccupied. He was faced with a big problem. Though this area was picturesque to look at, the rolling hills interfered with the television reception. My dad was shattered. His dream house conflicted with another dream of his. Yet with the belief that there is always a solution to every problem, he erected an even bigger pole at the end of the garden, one that could pick up the signals from the city, about a forty minute drive away.

The Flanagans had made their mark in this territory.

It wasn't long before some neighbors asked to be linked in, then more followed, and eventually my dad linked up most of the small community. I found it difficult to fathom that one small antenna at the back of my house could receive a signal from many miles away: a signal that is invisible to the naked eye and travels through buildings, in rain or shine, past fields, over roof tops and rolling hills faster than the speed of light. Then it continues through a network of cables buried beneath the ground into the living rooms of all who watch an identical television program at the same time.

I can still remember the lead up to Christmas, when all the children in the neighborhood gathered at my house to record our annual Christmas Show. We'd dress up, sing or mime our favorite song, read a poem, tell a story, or take part in a play. Miming was my forte. Sr. Ann had taught me well.

At three p.m. on Christmas Day, our show broadcast into the homes of everyone linked in. In multiple homes across the community, there were many emotions about this: children got excited, teenagers cringed, blushed or simply laughed, parents were entertained or bored, etcetera. The signal arrived at the same time to many homes and then transformed from something invisible into moving images, sound, color and light through their televisions.

Had I also transmitted a distress signal to the other side of the world, and my dad had somehow received it? Had the signal been transformed into images and sounds in his dreams? Was I imagining this? Or was this just some unexplainable parent-child connection, something to do with our DNA even? It made me wonder. The weird, wonderful and unexplainable tickled my curiosity. Communication was my wonderland. I often wondered if we send signals to one another the way we can with television and don't yet realize it.

There had to be something inside my body that could not only receive and transform signals into pictures and sounds in my head, but could also transmit them. There had to be something that I could not see that was common to every cell. Was there a commonality that gave cells the ability to "talk" to each other, both inside and out? My head was buzzing. This mental state reminded me of Dad's preoccupied look that I had witnessed so many years ago.

I am like Dad in so many ways, or so I've been told. Even my career path followed in his footsteps. I too was a creative thinker interested in color, movement, sound, vibration; I expressed this through art and design. New technology and science have a magnetic pull over me. It was by no coincidence that muted silence had steered me towards creativity, visual expression, and an interest outside the box for a reason. I believe inner wisdom did have a grand master plan because it was this path into the world of creativity where some of the answers I sought resided. I just didn't realize those lessons at the time.

I can still picture the daily trip to and from college and how this path had somehow been set to teach me something. Stepping off the 'Dart' at Pearce Street train station, the closest stop was at the back entrance to Trinity College, Ireland's haven of scholars. This, a 400 year old haven or breeding ground of academic learning and home to the famous *Book of Kells,* an illuminated manuscript created by the Celtic Monks of ca. 800 or slightly earlier. History and knowledge was difficult to avoid taking this path.

Through the back college gates I'd go, passing the seat of science, medicine, law, business, catching an eyeful of the refreshing green sports ground, via the great library of wisdom, onto a cobble stone pathway that radiated footsteps of famous scholars who had once walked there, then through Trinity's famous front archway, a meeting place and symbol of scholars and academics. And despite Trinity College not being my final destination, this route would become an every day occurrence over the next four years.

In contrast, I was headed to a world of paint, color and creative expression, to the National College of Art and Design which was about a fifteen minute walk from the train station. Someone had once told me that art was for stupid people; the path I was headed on was so far from this assertion. Located in the heart of the historical Liberties, Tomas Street where the scent of hops infiltrated the morning air from the Guinness factory next to my college. History tells that the art college grounds used to be part of the distillery, unique in design with the original smoke chimney still standing, old brewers vats linked to a network of colorful painted pipes that once carried Ireland's black gold—Guinness. Our unwritten dress code—to wear attire covered in paint of the colors of the rainbow, with an intense creative gaze, brush and sketchbook as tools, and a portfolio case to hold our painted moments captured in time.

Every evening on my way home I'd take a detour stopping off at Trinity's department of physics to pick up my next door neighbor and friend Luca. He was originally from France and had moved to Ireland to study his Ph.D. in laser physics, a branch of science that involves the behavior and properties of light and its interactions with matter. Just like sound, I would learn that light also had a hidden power—it too could move things.

Over time the other Ph.D. students jokingly began to call me an 'honorary member' of the physics group from my frequency of visits. I wonder what the nun who had once guided my career path might have thought about this. Indirectly I had made it to the science arena, to the most prestigeous university in Ireland. Regardless, my interest in science was growing. Many an evening was spent hanging out surrounded by the world of science as I waited for Luca to complete his daily laser experiments. My unconscious mind was like a sponge.

One day in particular I had a college project which baffled me. The brief was to answer 'What is blue?" except I wasn't allowed to answer this using paint or any other opaque substances. I turned to Luca for his scientific expertise. His answer would change how I perceived color thereafter.

Luca proceeded to explain the electromagnetic spectrum of light. He told me that the visible part of the spectrum is what the eyes see as color, and that so much more existed in our world that wasn't seen— there was an invisible world. That non-visible light had many attributes; it could be heard on the radio, used to see the body with ultrasound; dolphins communicate with it; we transmit and receive signals that we see and hear on our televisions, cell phones, computer and screens. The bumble bee is guided by it, so too are the birds; we use it for satellite systems on a planetery scale; we heat food in the microwave oven with it; alarm systems use it to detect movement and thermal heat; it gives us a suntan; it enables us to see soft bones and tissue using x-rays; we sterilize with it; we can mutate and destroy cells, cause cancer, destroy viruses, bacteria, pollute, and ultimately kill each other with it.

It was in this invisible world where my enemy resided. It was a place I was most definitely interested in exploring further. Luca had only scratched the surface.

Little did I know but I had only asked him to explain a small fraction of the spectrum. I was studying art and I hadn't once realized beforehand that light was color and so much more.

Luca had opened my eyes to what I could not see and what I had previously and so easily taken for granted. My environment both inside and out was literally an ocean of waves: radio waves, microwaves, infrared radiation, ultraviolet rays, x rays, and gamma rays. And like sound, the multitude of colors I saw were unique because each color had its own individual wave frequency. A "photon" is the scientific term for light, an individual packet of energy that travels from the sun to earth, moving in a wave-like pattern at the speed of light. This packet has both an electric and magnetic component, thus, that is why light is sometimes referred to as electromagnetic waves.

"The color red has a different wave-like pattern than the color blue," Luca said. "The wave frequency, wavelength, and energy content are what determines the color you see." I can still remember him saying that.

Unknowingly I had learned that anything living or nonliving that produces energy has an electrical or light frequency that vibrates. It fascinated me that a light source resided in almost everything, including me. Each was made up of infinite combinations of limitless vibrations;

our individual energy frequency fingerprints make us unique. Luca's conversation had been very significant that day; I just didn't know how much it was at the time.

Color absorbed my world; it permeated my creations, my thoughts, and the way I dressed. What I wore told of my zany or somber mood, and even my hair had its own unique story to tell. I even dreamed in bright, vivid color. But it hadn't always been that way. In early childhood blue had been my main attire; my sister so close in age most always got pink to wear and I the blue dress; Santa gave me dolls that always wore blue, my sister's dolls favored pink; and my uniform at high school, you guessed it, was dark blue. Paula and I were so close in age that rather than display any parental favoritism, we generally got the same style of clothes to wear from our parents, distinguishable only by our personally assigned color.

Eventually, as I grew older, blue would become one of my least favorite colors to wear. I rarely designed anything in blue except if specific to a design brief. The only time I wore this color was if I had to, if it was a gift, or if it had been handed down to me. In my teens, depending on my mood, my color preference swayed a lot towards wearing bright red. This color literally energized me. I was a rebel so red somehow gave me power. Black was its partner. But that was then and this is now. Red items are now hard to find in my wardrobe these days, quite the opposite from before. But on my path of healing, to my surprise, red craved a particular shade of green as its new partner. And instead of black furniture, it had to be white—white furniture with feature walls painted a particular shade of red and green, accessorized with red and green cushions, funky lamps, and bed linens. I can't imagine being surrounded by black couches and dark bookshelves today. I'd personally feel closed in. But back then I absolutely loved being surrounded by all things black, it was as if the darkness absorbed my nervous energy. And the colors I chose to wear or craved reflected my mood, frame of mind, and even my state of health.

Fashion and textile design was my chosen college major. It is ironic to think that making the outer shell more appealing gave me so much pleasure, as did interior design. With a background immersed in a wealth of history and Irish culture, the study of ancestral symbols and their meanings was a must on the curriculum, so was learning about the psychology of color. It fascinated me to learn that color can have a dramatic influence on how we feel, our mood, what we are thinking, our language, our appetite or thirst, and even on our health. It doesn't matter if color was something ingested, seen or imagined, it has a big influence.

I can still remember my first college field trip. Once a year the class would travel to the west of Ireland where we'd stay for a week, recording the environment. This rocky and barren part of the country is home to rare flora, set against the dramatic backdrop of cliffs and a steely gray wild ocean. Small whitewashed cottages, the kind taken straight from a tourist magazine, are dotted everywhere. White sprays from the turbulent waves try to crash above the huge cliff's edge. This place is truly remarkable, and not just for the budding artist or creative types. Its jewel shines even during the winter months, when cold, dampness, and the wind chill factor cut like knives. My breath smoked in front of my face, my hands froze without gloves, but the sunset over the ocean in icy temperatures would be the most colorful and memorable I'd ever encounter.

This day was particularly cold as we, the students, headed off in separate directions across the worn windswept rocky terrain. This was the site where the worst of the Great Irish Famine hit only a century before. The people of this region still show its wake—they are hardy and enduring. They are born survivors of this not so fertile and sparse land, a sea of gray bumps that can be seen for miles. Small rocks litter this terrain, illuminated by rock pools from recent rain glistening white in the low winter sun. Sunset was approaching. I sat on a makeshift piece of cardboard as protection from the elements—armed with paint, canvas, and memory cells ready to capture this moment.

Little did I know but nature had already decided to deliver the most amazing spectacle of color: red, orange, yellow, green-blue, purple, all the colors of the rainbow were getting ready to come out and play, then as if sucked away by the sun, darkness would absorb the colorful playtime. I thought of what Luca had told me about electromagnetic waves, and my imagination ran wild just thinking about the zillions of photons zigzagging around in the atmosphere, on the incoming waves from the sun that had created this unique show, a once-off, never-to-be-the-same-again spectacle and visual delight.

I slipped on my science cap to observe lazy washes of red painted across the sky, the laziest light in the visible spectrum. Their zigzag motion is the longest, their energy is lowest, and they travel a longer distance. As these red photons interacted with molecules such as water, air, dust particles, nitrogen, carbon, gases, vapors, etcetera, this caused them to vibrate, thus generating thermal heat. Red was in pursuit of yellow, hungry for green. Yellow light illuminates its positive rays in pursuit of its released neutral nucleus, blue. Blue light covers a shorter distance; its waves are shorter, its energy is higher. Blue light is magnetic. As blue photons enter the earth's atmosphere, some of the shorter waves are eliminated by air, and blue light scatters in all directions. I sat and watched the sky change color, knowing that as nature's movie unfolded before my eyes, so too did the electromagnetic atmosphere.

When the air is clear, the sunset will appear yellow, but when it is polluted with small particles, it will be red. Sunsets over the sea can appear to be more orange; that means there is more salt in the air. Today's spectacle was like a blood orange dissolving into the gray/bluish hues of the ocean.

Thankfully, the short winter day had come to an end as we headed back to our warm cottages for the evening. We'd chow down our evening meal, of which mine was closely monitored, and then we'd make our way to the local pub. In this neck of the country, the local pub was generally a small house in the heart of the village. It was hard to resist the large open fire and living room atmosphere during long, dark winter nights. Making a beeline to the cozy fireplace, I was surprised when I fell into a type of trance. The colors of the ambers and burning turf mesmerized me.

"Photons are everywhere," I thought as I sat watching the colors of the flames. But this was only a thought, one without action. Even though I had only recently found out about the existence of non-visible light, I was no different than a person walking past an incident on the street. This additional knowledge was passed off as something for the scientists, unrelated to me. It wouldn't enter my life as relevant until I came to realize that light influenced molecular behavior, infiltrated the food I ate, the clothes I wore, my body and mind, and more so my unconscious. If light can cause molecules to rotate or vibrate, generate heat, and cells to mutate and die, then it became my utmost interest to delve further into this vast invisible and unknown world.

I had never realized before that light could be so remarkable. It surprised me that I had taken it for granted all these years. I had never once stopped to think about it or even try to define it. It would take me nearly twenty years to realize this. Sadly, I had to end up facing a health crisis first. Regardless, from that day forth, every time I painted a sunrise or sunset, the ocean waves crashing off the Irish coast, or the various shades in the folds of fabric thereafter, photons literally entered the center of my mind.

"I am a light designer," I remember saying to Luca with a smile. Little did I know that this would eventually become my truth. The masterpiece I would end up painting would be to save my own life.

Many years had passed, and so too had time spent collecting as much information about my predicament as possible. The storage boxes in my apartment were growing as was the dust. Still on the hunt for answers, the modern day hunter-gatherer, the !Kung tribe caught my attention again. Not only did I find their sleeping patterns interesting, but also their beliefs about ill health and death. They believe that ill health or death manifests when the spirits shoot an invisible arrow in the direction of a person and that these invisible arrows can be stopped by their healing dance. Their healers dance around a fire until they are in a trance, the state that activates a powerful force they call "n/um". When in this state, they believe that they can heal whoever is sitting around the fire. It surprised me that these people didn't have the same technology as we do, yet they were aware of invisible arrows of light. I thought these invisible arrows might be non-visible light.

I wondered: does the tribe get a natural balance of *blue* and *yellow* light during the day and *yellow* and *red* light when they sit around the fire at night? Modern society uses artificial light, and there is nothing naturally balancing about it. What of the chemical cocktails on our tables? These people don't have the same ailments as people in modern society do; they are generally in good health. If their belief was true, then these invisible arrows affected both the body and brain.

I was intrigued. If light could cause molecules to change behavior in the external environment, then I hypothesized that the same could be true internally. This confirmed what I had learned in college: color can literally change your mood—a physical reaction occurs within upon seeing a color. It is the same with sound emulating from the radio.

Sometimes just hearing a song makes me feel sad, or other times it makes me want to get up and dance—I can literally feel the music, an internal shift happens within.

The entire human body is designed to respond to electrically charged and coded messages that establish health, restore harmony, and bring about healing. The brain operates on electrical currents, and the nervous system uses electrical currents to send and receive signals. The balance and interaction of sodium and potassium form an electrical charge that helps carry food (in), fluid, and waste in and out of cell walls—the electrical charge is light. Chemically, electrolytes such as sodium, chloride, potassium, and bicarbonate are essential for cell communication as these substances in solution have the capacity to conduct electricity.

"Literally, my body is swimming in an ocean of light," I thought. "Light is essential for communication on a cellular level—essential for survival."

This would turn my journey down a scientific route which found that every disease has a frequency, and that certain frequencies can prevent the development of disease and that others could destroy diseases. Substances of higher frequency will destroy diseases of lower frequency. Basically every cell in the body vibrates at its own frequency fingerprint, and group of cells that make up bodily systems have their own frequencies as well. An organ is composed of cells of similar vibrations that have gathered to form that organ. Larger, more complicated systems, which themselves are contained within even larger and more complex structures all vibrate.

Even the energy vibration emanating from a potato plant is different than that of a tomato plant. That is what makes them different. It's the vibration, the frequency, the light. All living things share this commonality—that is light.

My body is designed to detect different stimuli or frequencies emanating from both my internal and external worlds—light, sound, chemicals, heat, and pressure. Electrical signals that fire off faster than the speed of light cluster around the entire body. The observer cannot see this but can sometimes feel it. It does all of this without one having even to think about it. Depending on the frequency, the body will respond accordingly to the signals it receives through the senses. Particular energy fingerprints received through our eyes, ears, nose, mouth, and skin that our brain interprets tell us about our world. Our eyes perceive color, our ears absorb sounds vibrations, our nose and mouth receive chemical signals, and our skin responds to heat and pressure.

Living organisms have measurable frequencies on various levels, and the entire human body, even down to the cellular level, is no exception. Cells regenerate all the time. The hardest working cells have the shortest lifespan. Eye cells have been recorded to take just two days to regenerate, the small intestine just one week or less, taste buds about ten to fourteen days, colon cells approximately three to four weeks, the liver six weeks, olfactory neurons (in the nose) thirty to forty days. Eyelashes and eyebrows can take up to two months, and red blood cells take four months.

Scientific research shows that there is a distinct difference in frequencies between a healthy human body and an unhealthy one. Research shows that the average frequency of a healthy human body during the daytime is 62 to 68Hz (62 – 68 wave cycles per second). When the frequency drops, the immune system is stressed. For example, if the frequency drops to 58Hz, cold and flu symptoms manifest; at 55Hz candida takes hold; and at 42Hz cells can mutate into cancer. They discovered that illness, infection, and varying diseases can only exist at particular frequencies which are always within their own definite range. Illness or infection is the result of normal frequency patterns increasing (from long to shorter wavelengths), known as "hyper" ones in medical terms ("hyper" means high). When the frequency decreases (short to longer wavelengths) it is known as "hypo", which in medical terms means low.

Many pollutants have low frequencies and cause the body's healthy frequencies to be lowered and weakened. Processed or canned foods contain zero frequency and tend to lower the healthy body frequency towards degenerative disease. In a study, scientists took two young men, each with a 66Hz frequency. One of the men held a cup of coffee, and his frequency dropped to 58Hz in three seconds. The other man was asked to drink his coffee. His frequency dropped to 52Hz in three seconds. Simply by drinking a hot cup of coffee, the second man's body became susceptible to colds and flu, candida, and many other conditions. If coffee could have that effect on the body just by smelling its aroma or holding a cup of coffee, then I was curious to find out more about what other food or drink did on a cellular level.

Food contains molecular compounds of amino acids, various chemicals, and complex carbohydrate chains. Each has its own unique vibration or frequency. It is the vibrations of nutrients that raise the vibrations of the body's tissues. Pesticide and chemically-treated fruits and vegetables, as well as meat or animals contaminated with antibiotics and growth hormones, have chaotic vibratory oscillations that can derail their benefit to the body's nutritional energy needs.

Fritz-Albert Popp, a theoretical biophysicist in Germany, found that molecules in cells responded to certain frequencies, and that a range of light vibrations created an array of frequencies in other molecules throughout the body. He theorized that light controls everything in the cell. His research confirmed that living cells emit small bursts of light; that cells both radiate light and absorb it. He claims that the storage time of light is relative to the quality of the cell. This means that a healthy cell stores light the longest, whereas an unhealthy cell will release the light in less time.

According to Popp, the most basic sub-molecular component of the human body is made up of particles of light called biophotons. These travel at the speed of light and make up the electromagnetic patterns found in every living organism. He found that this field of frequency oscillations provides the energetic switch-boarding behind every cellular function, including DNA/RNA. DNA is made up of a salt (sodium). Sodium is one of the body's major electrolytes and a conductor of electromagnetism. He also found that the light content in food deteriorates, alters or is damaged when it is cooked or frozen.

If cells, organs, and glands have a weak vibration or the light is dim, they cannot carry out their processes properly. The same applies if the vibration or light is too strong or too intense. When these processes are disrupted for any extended period of time, chances of illness and/or death are heightened. Diseases manifest when this natural balance of vibration is disrupted or out of whack. It is when this vibration ceases in our vital organs such as the heart, brain or lungs that we die. When the light is dim, the body will adjust its internal functions for survival. Every disease is a reaction originating from the inside out.

Yet most of us focus on fixing the symptoms or the effects, even when a deeper path to the cellular problem has been revealed. Our body is designed to heal and protect us at all costs—the physical symptoms are designed to bring our awareness of the problem to reveal the path to resolve it. Without the balance of free-flowing electrical impulses, the body becomes vulnerable to false messages or signals. These false messages or signals also emanate from us into our outside world to cause disharmony. These are reactions which can be positive and give us life, or they have the potential of negativity causing us harm.

Invisible light is transferred back and forth all the time. Sometimes lines can get crossed, blocked, broken, or they can mutate or fade to create an illusion of nothing more than smoke, mirrors, blocks of distortions, and confusion. Light is key to survival because without it our own worlds would fall into disarray and die out. These vibrations have a fundamental and literal impact on everything. The food we eat, the colors we see, the aromas we smell, the emotions we feel, the surfaces we touch, the thoughts we have—diseases, viruses, toxins, and basically everything that has energy has its own unique frequency. This is what is sensed and what the body uses to communicate, protect, digest, heal, and replicate. Sadly most of us only start to listen to the body's messages when life hangs in the balance and we have no other option but to act.

Thinking about my dad's "telepathy" about my reactions, I wondered, "Is there an antenna/transmitter located in the human body?" If I found an answer to this, then maybe I had a chance of finding the wizard orchestrating both internal and external communication. This exquisite communicator had the ability to send, receive, alter and adapt information at the speed of light. Could I alter the communications to heal myself of reactions?

"Dad's dream," I thought. "Could that be a clue?"

After all, it was through a dream that he apparently received my signal—through a movie playing in his mind's eye. That a dream might simply be an internal television, displaying invisible information received through the senses, which was then converted into images, sounds, colors, and thoughts inside the head intrigued me.

Are dreams more than we give them credit for?

Are they another way for the brain to recognize or make sense of this forever changing world—a way to make sense of the invisible information or signals it receives? By becoming aware of some of these invisible factors, might this quiet the mind and body?

Could the pineal gland, the regulator of sleep/wake cycles, be the answer to this? The pineal gland is sensitive to seasons and annual events. It sits in darkness deep in the center of the brain, yet it is sensitive to light. Non-visible light? Its position is behind the root of the nose, between the left and right hemispheres of the brain, and behind and just above the pituitary gland (the master gland). The pineal is the first gland to form in the fetus, and it has a profuse blood flow, second only to the kidneys. Therefore, it must be of great importance. There was a feeling in my bones that I should delve into this a bit deeper. It was time to put my science cap on again.

I found that the hormone melatonin is secreted by the pineal gland to regulate the daily body clock and the sleep/wake cycle (Appendix: Melatonin). Research shows that the pineal gland has the highest calcium concentration of any normal soft tissue in the body which calcifies with age. Calcification is the process in which calcium salts build up in soft tissue, causing the tissue to harden. Pineal calcification, which is a natural occurrence, over time can affect the brain's ability to function and perform daily life tasks (Appendix:: Calcium). (see Appendix at the back of this book for a more detailed discussion of pineal calcification and fluoride)

I was intrigued to discover that science now supports the idea that this gland is nature's first eye. Under the microscope, the pineal is formed of light-sensitive cells similar to the retina of the eyes. They also discovered piezoelectric crystals in the pineal gland. Piezo crystals are material that has the ability to generate electric charges when their shape is compressed, twisted or distorted. The deformation of the crystal shifts its positive and negative charge, thus creating an external electric field. This is called piezoelectricity. This means that this type of crystal can act like a transmitter or receiver.

"My body has its own built in antenna system," I thought.

Research also showed that the pineal crystal had a striking resemblance to crystals found in the inner ear, in the bones, teeth, intestines, and in connective tissue such as ligaments, cartilage, and tendons. This probably explains why credence is given to a *gut feeling* or that *I feel something in my bones* is the truth. Piezoelectricity can also be found in the trachea, aorta, silk, wood and ivory. One of the earliest types of radio, a mineral crystal was made to resonate with incoming radio waves. Six piezo crystals are placed under the strings of an electric guitar to convert the sound wave into electric energy, which is amplified many times before reaching the ear. This can also work in reverse. For example, when electric nerve pulses hit the piezo crystals in the intestines, they move and distort to convert the electrical energy into mechanical energy to move its contents.

The pineal gland connects all the dots as an organ that can send, receive, alter and adapt information at the speed of light. It has ties with DNA and access to absolutely every cell in the body via the blood. Its sensitivity to light points to only one thing: that it must be the control center to receive, decipher, convert, and regulate photon frequencies (electromagnetic waves) to maintain good health and, if out of balance, it can upset the transfer of information to many cells across the organism.

Russian scientist Dr. Garjajev suggested that communication isn't limited to inside or between one cell and another but that organisms use "light" to "talk" to other organisms. He says that this could explain telepathy and extra sensory perception. In 1923, while experimenting with communication between plants, he discovered that two onion plants communicated with each other by ultraviolet light—photons. "Cells communicate both electromagnetically and chemically and create biochemical pathways that interconnect with all functions of the body," reported Dr. Garjajev.

I can still recall the day when my research led to a study by the U.S. military. In this experiment they collected DNA in the form of leukocytes (white blood cells) from participants, placing the cells into a chamber so that they could measure electrical changes, if any. The participants were placed in a different room away from the collected DNA, instructed to watch video clips designed to elicit various emotional responses. The experiment concluded that at the exact same moment the participant showed emotional peaks or valleys, surprisingly their DNA in the other room exhibited an identical response. The electrical peaks and valleys of both the DNA sample and the participant matched. They stopped the test after the participant had been placed fifty miles away from their DNA concluding that they achieved the exact same result; electrical peaks and valleys from both the participant and their DNA sample, with no lag time between transmissions. Time and distance didn't matter.

This study got me wondering. Had Dad simply picked up on my white blood cells in trauma? That they had somehow communicated what I was feeling to him?

Could the pineal gland be the key to my body's communication system and thus my health? Could it be the key to the signals my body was over-reacting to? Could it be the key to living a normal life, without being in mortal danger every second? I believed I had found the key piece to the puzzle of my health.

"What is blue?" had taken me on a journey I hadn't anticipated. And it was about to get even more interesting.

I was dumbfounded when I discovered some research that showed melatonin is suppressed in certain frequencies of blue light.

Blue light? If melatonin is suppressed in certain frequencies of blue light, then this would mean that the upper gastrointestinal tract could be left unprotected during melatonin suppression.

Could this mean that certain blue lighting or surroundings, blue food coloring, consistently wearing blue-colored clothing, eating off blue plates or in front of a blue computer screen during food intake can suppress the release of melatonin in the upper part of the gastrointestinal tract during the day? Therefore, blue light and color can suppress appetite, induce a state of immunodepression and reduce antioxidant properties which protect nuclear and mitochondrial DNA.

Blue food is a rare occurrence in nature, which would explain the importance of melatonin release during digestion. When the hunter-gatherer ancestors were foraging for food, anything blue, purple or black was taken as a "color warning sign" of potentially lethal food. What surprises me is that more and more blue-colored food is marketed to children today. Research shows that some people can have an allergic reaction to food coloring. Brilliant blue FCF 133 may be dangerous to asthmatics; it may cause a hyperactive response and may affect people who cannot tolerate aspirin.

Could this response just be part of the body's natural protection process to deal with an excess of blue photon frequencies in its attempt to restore balance to over-activity in the brain and nervous system due to vulnerability in the upper digestive tract as its means to survive?

It would make sense that the *blue* end of the spectrum (high-energy and shorter wavelengths) must play more of a role in electrical processes of nerve cell communication. And that the *red* end of the spectrum (low-energy and longer wavelengths) must play more of a role in temperature (thermal), mechanical, and chemical processes. Research showed that the color blue stimulated glands, organs, and the nervous system (sympathetic branch), whereas red relaxed them (parasympathetic branch).

To activate the pineal gland, both the pineal gland and the pituitary gland must vibrate in unison. This can be achieved through meditation, deep relaxation, or hypnosis. I would also become more conscious of blue light and other colors, such as what I ingested or drank on a regular basis. I began to listen to Solfeggio frequency 528 Hz everyday, the frequency known to repair DNA—this I believe can help to reset the genetic switchboard.

I had learned that each color can influence behavior on a molecular level when combined with the conditions of the environment such as air, fluid, moisture, gas, heat, cold, pressure, pollutants, chemicals, toxins, bacteria, and even emotion. Just recognizing how food changes its natural color when it is cooked or frozen told me this.

Food I COULD eat was now under scrutiny. This included food preparation and storage—boiling, frying, grilling, roasting, freezing, etcetera. With the addition of these added influences, the molecular behavior of the raw or unprocessed food/drink is altered, thus the body and immune system react to this new altered frequency in a different way.

I began to introduce more live, fresh, unprocessed, raw food into my diet. I also changed when I ate certain foods which had a similar frequency to particular organs and bodily functions using the color of the food/toxin as a guide.

Not only did this preserve light properties as nature had intended, it also minimized the amount of labels I had to read on a regular basis. Gradually, over time as the internal environment improved, so too did my pineal gland, as nightmares or flashbacks during specific time-triggers dissolved.

The answer to my college project "What is Blue?" was this;
  Blue $= C (G + B) - \textbf{\textit{R}} + M (R + B) - \textbf{\textit{G}}$

I had created a formula outside of the 'normal' way of thinking.

  C=Cyan
  G=Green
  B=Blue
  R=Red
  M=Magenta

Appendix: Making Sense
24 hour cycle – Peak energy/activity of organs
The Effects of Visible Light on the Body
Frequencies/Wavelengths in Association with the Body
Raw Food versus Cooked Food

25

Passage to the Heart

"Start by doing what's necessary; then do
what's possible; and suddenly
you are doing the impossible."

St. Francis of Assisi

Four months had passed since I chose to follow my heart and take a passage into unknown territory in search of answers for my allergies. Within a short space of time, instinctively I knew that my mind, body, heart, and soul had been touched and profoundly altered forever. It was time to test my efforts. The medical response wouldn't be what I had expected.

"I think we've made a mistake," my doctor said on the other end of the phone. This was something I hadn't been expecting.

"I'm sorry...your blood test results...I mean...they..." I listened intently to this familiar trusted voice while looking at Ann, my boss. Nearly a year had passed since I started in this company. Ann and I had become really good colleagues and friends. Her unflagging support had made all the difference working among others in the office. I had been blessed since the day I disclosed my medical history to her, lucky that she understood my struggles with compassion. She had suggested that I make this call during work hours, especially for these particular results. This time I wasn't alone. But this moment came attached with an awkwardness I was still getting used to—that of accepting help.

Today, Ann watched with anticipation as I nodded in response to my doctor's voice on the other end of the phone, my eyes fixed on her to indirectly include her in this conversation. She genuinely cared about my well-being—unlike some of the other bosses I had worked for. With her reservoir of caring waiting on-hand, I could feel her shoulder's willingness to take some of the burden off my soul. This meant a lot to me, especially today as it would turn out that these particular blood test results had taken a lifetime to reach me.

"Can you come into my practice for another blood test now?" my doctor asked, hoping to be face-to-face within an hour. Disbelief was in her voice—this unusual shift in tone rang clear. I was used to precision and directness from her but I heard nothing but uncertainty—doubt—and urgency in her voice on this particular morning.

"What do you mean exactly?" I asked, confirming whether I had heard her right. I had already predicted this, but the depth of my soul insisted on hearing it again.

By now the room and the people in it had gone on pause—three other colleagues had swiveled their chairs around to fix their eyes on me. I grinned. The slight hum of the computers circling the perimeter acted as the buffer for my increasingly inquisitive voice. Again time froze—as if we had all tuned directly into the now, dialed in perfect unison—fixated. Thoughts of the future didn't exist, nor did the past—there was only this moment.

"I think we might have gotten your blood mixed up," my doctor said, pausing for a moment. "The results are negative."

If I didn't know better, she sounded as if these results were bad—an error or a mistake even. I held my breath. My heart began to flurry in a way I didn't remember encountering before.

"Negative," I repeated, knowing that in medical terms this means that a condition or disease wasn't detected. This was the only negative I truly wanted in my life and now that I got it, I really didn't know how to receive it—I was a total novice to medical negatives. We both lapsed into stunned silence over the phone.

As I listened to the silence, a volcano of long-forgotten sensations began to bubble up from my core. These lessons of the past, caught under the rocks of life, began to loosen—to break free. It felt as if learned behavior, habits or routines formulated over time which once limited flow were melting, losing rigidity. Possibility had opened its eyes in a slow awakening.

"I am at work now…I can't come during office hours," I said, disappointed that I would not be able to nip all doubt in the bud with a visit. I had waited a lifetime for this. But! There always seemed to be a "but" or additional conditions when I wanted something really badly.

I took a breath to savor the word "negative". As the realization that I might have succeeded began to sink in, permeating every cell in my body, my unconscious had begun to smile from inside out. The corners of my mouth wanted to curve upward. But in this context, responsibility and respect rapidly broke through. Medical protocol— whatever that might be had no precedent.

What was to come next? I didn't know.

How could I? I had little or no reference to a life without allergies. And I had definitely no reference point for a doctor telling me that I was normal—normal like everyone else. No allergies!

"Can you book me in for an early morning appointment...It has to be before I start work," I said, keen to get this cleared up as soon as possible. I wanted to drop everything and leave the office right there and then, but I couldn't. I had work commitments.

I had to be responsible.

"Don't go eating peanuts now," my doctor stressed, as if worried I'd lunge straight into doing this before seeing her. The thought had crossed my mind, but only for a brief moment. Eating peanuts was something I couldn't do on my own. My friends would most definitely never agree to watch me do it, my parents would come after me if the peanut didn't get there first, and my doctor would...well...I didn't know. All I knew was that there would be a lot of very upset people if I took this risk without medical supervision. Plus, risking my life wasn't worth it.

"What, next week is the earliest you can squeeze me in?" I asked in dismay, knowing that waiting for this appointment would be the longest wait of my life—a sentence.

A week seemed like a lifetime. It seemed to me that when your life depends on something so much, time goes askew—it speeds up, slows down, or simply freezes. The sense of distance appears to be the same—something is so close, within reach, yet so far away. To have made it this far and then to have to follow the medical procedure frustrated me, but I knew this was imperative.

"Go now!" exclaimed Ann, catching me off guard. "Go on...what are you waiting for?" she continued. I hadn't noticed that Ann had already gathered my belongings, and she now ushered me out of the office. It was a first that being ousted for anything to do with my allergies was done with an embrace. For me, it was as if she had just fired a gun at the starting line, I moved in positive motion as people cheered me on, genuinely wanting me to reach the finish line—to reach my goal—to triumph.

Over the next week déjà vu would strike twice-fold—two more blood tests—two identical sets of results.

"There is no way in the world human error could have occurred three times," I thought during the second, almost word-for-word phone conversation with my doctor. Again, Ann and three other colleagues sat within earshot. When the third blood test came back, I decided to receive these results in person. I couldn't sit back and do nothing, especially when three messages told the same story.

"Michelle, according to these three pieces of paper in my hand, each result shows that you are normal—someone without allergies," my doctor said, shaking her head in disbelief. "I took your blood myself…I sent it to the lab…and blood tells the truth. Error has to be ruled out, especially when each test was performed at different times over a three week period."

I smirked in quiet triumph.

"Normal, like everyone else."

These words replayed over and over again in my mind. I hadn't heard these words to describe me ever before. I doubted I would ever hear them again.

"I'm not sure what to do now," my doctor admitted. I appreciated her honesty and humility. She continued, "I couldn't find any precedent to follow…I even asked my fellow colleagues. Frankly I have never heard of Anaphylaxis disappearing like this before, especially when you've had it for such a long time, and as an adult. I know you have been focusing on this for the last few months…but I thought your mission was impossible…these results have really surprised me." I listened, quietly smiling from the inside out.

The results had spoken.

Deep down, I knew that I had triumphed over what was once believed impossible. I knew without a doubt that I had succeeded. I was humbled that my inner wisdom had blessed me on this journey so far, yet I had absolutely no idea what else was in store.

We both paused for a moment, looking around the room while deep in thought. I covered my mouth with one hand. I looked to heaven for some inspiration. I was dazed, still processing this new information, even as possibility brought forth a flood of ideas. The most obvious was plucked off the train of thoughts to declare its rightful space.

"Can you write a referral letter for one of Sydney's known immunologists, please?" I asked, telling my doctor his name, mentioning that he was also a professor, and that I saw him about ten years before when I first arrived in Australia. It had been a daunting time then, to be told that the peanut allergy would be with me for life—that there was literally nothing I could do about it. He knew my case well and so too did the hospital where he had his consulting room. The hospital was located in my suburb, where I'd accumulated a long record of emergency room visits. I was registered as an Anaphylactic in the area. I was well known as a frequent E.R. visitor in need of life-saving allergy treatment. It seemed fitting that this particular chapter in my life should find some resolution on familiar territory.

"Of course I will write a referral letter for you, but you must be prepared. There can be about a six month wait to see specialists of such a caliber," she replied, trying not to squash my enthusiasm as she struck letters on her keyboard. I felt humbled that she had acknowledged how far I had come on this journey and that she was sympathetic that I might have to wait for a few months to cross the finish line.

"Um, I understand. I don't want to sound cocky, but I think when he sees the three negative results associated with my medical history, he will want to see me straight away," I said, smiling.

Reaching the goal I had aspired to achieve felt surreal. This altered reality was still forming new neural pathways—a lifetime of the word "incurable" took time to fade. I had reached a point when "incurable" and "curable" met in debate; instinct and belief vied for attention while trust and the essence of self were sitting in the transit lounge. I had nothing to compare to this. Living a life with, and then without Anaphylaxis was unheard of.

My predictions had been spot on. Curiosity had touched the immunologist and it was only three weeks before we were sitting face-to-face. Ten years had come and gone between us. I had been in my twenties when I saw him last. So much debris and turbulence had passed under the bridge of life since then. "But enough of the past," said the voice inside my head. "This is about the now and steps for the future." I desperately needed to know the truth. Not just for me, but for absolutely everybody I knew or didn't know who had been impacted directly or indirectly in some way or another by this condition. My family, partners, friends, acquaintances, teachers, bosses, colleagues, groups, communities, industries, manufacturers, businesses, governments, countries, and ultimately the world had all been touched by the hand of Anaphylaxis.

This was HUGE, especially the next and more immediate course of action. The final and most necessary act would also place me directly in the line of fire. I needed to pass the test of a food challenge, such as to eat peanuts in a controlled hospital setting. That was the only way to validate the blood test results.

"You don't have to do this—there are huge risks involved," the immunologist said, trying to stave off the inevitable. Finding the truth behind these three pieces of paper had my whole life's quest attached to it. If a food challenge was the only way, I was prepared to put my life on the line. For the first time I had been told that I was normal like everyone else. I had yearned for this all my life. I wasn't going to leave any stone unturned in making sure this allergy free result was real.

I said, "It's not about whether I can eat peanuts or not. It's about my whole life...I have to do this. Proving it in a medically controlled environment is the only real chance I have to reveal the truth...to reveal that the last few months have been worth it. My medical slate needs to be rewritten," I presented my case repeatedly and forcefully, and, at last, the immunologist agreed to the food challenge.

The battleground had been set.

"Okay, let me organize this with the Intensive Care Unit (ICU)," he said.

Two weeks would pass without word.

Finally I got the call I'd been waiting for. Again, I was at work.

"You are being admitted on Monday," said the nurse responsible for hospital admissions early on Friday morning. "Please get your affairs in order." In the same breath, she told that I'd probably be a week away from work, so I should let my employer know. Her words really brought home the danger of what I was about to do. For a brief moment I felt unnerved—uncertain, confused even. Her instruction had delivered two conflicting messages; one that I'd still be around in a week's time; the other that I wouldn't.

Even though I was expecting this pending hospital admission, having the date set shook me.

The final battle was in sight.

The countdown to a meeting with demons on the frontline had begun. I had a weekend to get my affairs in order.

A lot had to be done.

As usual I met my friends on Friday night, but this one would turn into an absolute blur like many forgotten nights of the past—drinking, partying, and having as much fun as I possibly could. Acting out to the max was an understatement.

This frenzy would infect most of my weekend. There was no one to hold my hand, to let me know that it would be okay, or to ground me. Nobody can prepare you for what I was about to do. Some might have said that I was trancing out or irresponsible at the time, but I didn't care what others thought. Despite my family being a great support, it didn't help that they were there and I was here.

I had received a phone call confirming the date, time, and finances associated with hospital admission. That was it. Similar to dealing with the aftermath of an anaphylactic reaction, no trained professional had been assigned to help me face the biggest source of trauma in my life. Imagine having to face your absolute worst and most intense nightmare on your own. There was no expert to help me through the emotional turmoil associated with facing death—facing what I had been told to avoid all my life. I was challenging learned survival strategies that had spanned a lifetime. I was about to take my very first step on my own moon.

I did what any normal person would do under the circumstances. Party central went wild. I didn't want the next few days to end—who would in this situation? I stayed out as much as I possibly could. I was single, no-one waited for me at home. The expression 'burn the candle at both ends' became an understatement. I didn't want to sleep. The fear of "missing out" had gone into overdrive. My friends did their best to keep me company over the weekend but eventually I found myself totally alone on Sunday night. All the emotions under the sun had come out to play that weekend—laughter, sadness, fear, confusion, doubt, love, anger, guilt, loneliness, courage—you name it, I felt it. Peace and reflection would eventually come.

I took out my journals to read while propping the pillow behind my back for added support and comfort.

The showdown was in a few hours.

Who would have believed that it had only taken a few months to journey back to my beginning and even further? Not one red blood cell floating around in my body had existed when I took the first leg of this journey into my allergies only four months ago. These fresh red blood cells had never encountered this enemy before; placed under the microscope, this blood had reported back to science that it did not recognize this enemy. It was because of this I was here, sitting on the verge of the unknown—about to say goodbye to a lifelong enemy and partner. I was waiting in position in the birth canal—my passage to nirvana, to a new life. Déjà vu of my first birth had come full circle, for each beginning is the start of a journey to another beginning.

Like every newborn, I had arrived naked from the depths of warm fluid into what I would later learn to call air. I took my first breath for survival and instinctively blinked my eyes to protect them against the bright new light illuminating the space in the elevator shaft. Foreign particles floated in the air. I naturally blinked again to wash them out. The gentle echoes of a heartbeat and the melodic gurgles of digestion were all but a distant memory of the last nine months. Time then meant nothing. But it would later. Cold and wet, my skin was wrapped in a strange texture, something I had never felt before. This came as a label; blue for boys, pink for girls—yellow for the unknown. As a newborn, my sense of touch was amplified as was my sense of smell. Nature had heightened these particular senses above the others for survival, to help me to move around, to learn about the strange unknown world I had just entered. Therefore, under extreme stress such as the task just around the corner I would remember to breathe, to take a breath, to feel new sensations—for the senses of smell and touch had once been my primary allies when I first entered a world of the unknown.

I had learned that even before my arrival, my existence had its challenges; my blood was incompatible with one of my creators, positive red could clash with negative red at anytime. The recent blood tests showed that the fight was no more. At the time I was born, food manufacturing processes were becoming more mainstream. That meant more toxins and more work for my immune system. My first arrival was unexpected and premature—a spontaneous preterm birth, they call it. Could a battle between positive red and negative red have triggered an early arrival? And where was the cuddle hormone? I pushed my mum away for days, weeks and even the months that would follow?

I entered the world in a birthday suit covered from head to toe in skin, a sensory organ that can detect touch or pressure, heat or cold, and pain. This is a sense I knew from when I had been in the womb, the place where I had just come from. From that moment onward this outer shell would unknowingly and continuously send information to my brain about my sense of self, other people, and the environment around me. Every time I touched or was touched would form the boundaries around the outer layer of my being.

I would learn that hugs bring love, trust, a sense of oneness, and they offer comfort through times of difficulty. Hugs are a gift and built-in security blanket of warmth. They welcome the cuddle hormone which keeps stress at bay. One size fits all. Without touch, love and trust filter through the outer veneer, leaving a type of coldness, loneliness, pain, and insecurity within. Embracing self when at my most vulnerable would be remembered. Touch connects to a felt sense, to a sensation within, a raw primal feeling (love, hurt, fear, anger). Creating energy in motion (e-motion) under the surface is guaranteed. The very things we touch provoke an emotional reaction. We may not know what that reaction is; however; there it is guaranteed that, once touched, an emotional feeling will follow.

I had learned that our DNA changes shape according to the feelings or emotions in its environment. Science discovered that intense positive emotion such as love, appreciation, and gratitude causes DNA to relax, such that the strands unwind and grow longer. That intense negative emotion such as anger, fear, stress, frustration or aggression causes DNA strands to wind up or tighten, thus switching 'off' many of the DNA codes. For this, I knew that a positive emotional state during the biggest test of my life was crucial.

Over the next hour that Sunday night before my hospital admission, I spent some time creating a touch anchor linked to a positive desired state to help in the moment of challenge. I knew that success depended on my emotional state, and I remembered a class I once had about the body and emotions. I used this to prepare for my challenge.

I can still recall my teacher's words when he was teaching us about posture and how it can affect our emotions.

"Okay everybody, I'd like you all to put your book down for a moment and try the following exercise," he said.

"While sitting on your chair, move your upper torso downward so that your chest rests on your upper thighs, flop your arms by your sides, touch the floor, and pretend that your whole body is limp, like a rag doll," I remember listening to his instructions as we comically mastered our floppy rag doll posture.

"Now from that same position, I want you to GET EXCITED!" he said with a louder, uplifting tone. Spurts of laughter, disbelief, and surprise filled the classroom as we all failed dismally to express excitement while the body was slumped down, floppy and deflated. It was incredible.

We were then asked to stand up straight, put our shoulders back, and be as alert and wide awake as possible. But in this instance…"Now feel depressed and down from this position," he instructed. Again we failed. It was interesting to see how much posture had an influence on a person's emotional state. If I felt depressed or down thereafter, I simply observed and changed my posture accordingly to shift any unwanted emotional states.

I pondered, "If posture can influence how I express my emotions, then any emotions picked up from the environment must also influence how the body holds itself so as to be able to carry the emotion. This would also affect bodily functions and, more importantly, could be an advantage to remember to shift posture if an intense negative emotion ever tried to take hold."

On the eve of the biggest day of my life working out a few battle strategies offered comfort. But that said, I thought of my family. They must be worried sick on the other side of the world. And even though I had spoken with my family on the phone earlier, I felt the need to write my parents a note.

Letter to my parents written the night before the final battle:

Dear Mum and Dad

I know that you really wanted to be with me in the morning when I eat peanuts in hospital. But, my heart has been telling me that the stress may be too much for all of us to handle. I understand that you would travel to the other end of the earth to stand by me, especially when I face the biggest challenge of my life. But, to be honest, my gut tells me that this final battle has to be fought alone.

Rest assured I have three blood test results that show I am no longer allergic. And my immunologist, who was surprised to see the results, will be by my side every step of the way, especially when I take my first bite. I want you to know that I've taken every precaution imaginable to stay safe. And please trust me when I tell you that this step is necessary for an answer. I hope you understand that by going through with this, contrary to everyone telling me not to, I do so only because I really need to know the truth.

It is 3 a.m., and I am still wide awake. I should feel anxious but instead I am relieved the light at the end of the tunnel is near. I am so close to finding out if all the steps I took over the last few months have ended this chapter. The blood test results say so.

You have both been my towers of strength and no words could ever thank you for that, especially when I told you about my quest to find a way to overcome this burden. I can't even try to imagine the worry I must have put you through, now and before. But you have always been there for me, no matter what. And even though sometimes you did not understand why I chose to take this road less traveled, I did so remembering your words: "Be careful, stay safe, and we love you".

I can't help but think of everything that has happened in my life. Would I have reached this moment if it weren't for the difficult situations, the people I have met, and the countries I have traveled to? I certainly would not have learned what I know today, especially if I didn't have your understanding, encouragement, support, and most important of all, your love.

I want you to know that I love you more than anything in this world. And because of you, I have the courage to take my first baby steps into an unknown world, to the place I know will set my soul free.

Love always,

Michelle

"Please send me someone to hold my hand when I face my demons," were the last words I wrote into my journal before I drifted off to sleep.

The doorbell rang. Andrew had arrived to take me to the hospital. I can still remember taking a final look around my apartment as I closed the door. I knew that life as I knew it might never be the same again.

He put my overnight bag in the back of the car, looking at me but saying nothing. Our facial expressions accompanied with a hug, was enough to communicate how we felt. Verbal expression was replaced by a now familiar sense of surreal—numbness I had become accustomed to what was attached to the unknown. I was connected to something I did not know yet—to what my mind was still working out. I really didn't know how to feel, and understandably so.

"I'm getting engaged," Andrew said, to break the silence.

"What?" I replied, not even sure he had said something.

"Yes! I pick up the ring once I drop you off," he replied.

Even though this announcement may have been a shock under any other circumstances, I was genuinely happy for him.

I had come a long long way in the year and a half that passed since we broke up. Andrew knew that. He also knew that today was as good a time as ever to tell me this happy news. I knew that any upset I might have had over it would only tell me that I hadn't let go of my past. I wasn't upset, and I had let go.

We spoke for a little about the ring, and then Andrew turned the radio on to catch the early morning show.

Déjà vu struck as the radio sent me a deep and private message, just as it did when my parents were on their way to the hospital that early February morning to deliver me—when the words of a particular song stood out:

"And through it all she offers me protection—a lot of love and affection…" I listened as Robbie Williams sang this very fitting song "Angels". The journey to the hospital and all thoughts and fear about what I was about to do next dissolved into this lullaby about angels.

It comforted me to believe that the angels were sending me a message—I wasn't alone—they were protecting and loving me.

"Michelle, we are going to have to cancel," said my immunologist on the other end of my mobile phone.

"Sorry what did you say? I am only five minutes from the hospital," I replied in disbelief. He couldn't cancel. I had spent the last few days and a lifetime preparing for this. Cancelling this food challenge would surely leave emotional scars.

"I checked with hospital catering—they don't have any peanuts in the kitchen," he explained.

"Can you not just go to the local shop and buy some?" I asked in disbelief. Cancelling a food challenge because the hospital didn't have any peanuts which are literally found everywhere?

"What's going on?" Andrew entered in. "Do you want me to stop on the way to buy some?"

"You know that you don't have to do this," the immunologist said again.

"But, I do…please, I really want to do this, especially now that I am so ready for it," I replied. "We are literally driving into the hospital car park now. I will see you in a few minutes."

We continued our conversation face-to-face. It took some more convincing to get a go ahead—but then a feast of the once forbidden was to begin. A nurse was sent to the shop to buy some peanuts, and I made my way to the intensive care ward.

Andrew waved goodbye.

26

The Beginning of an End
to another Beginning

"Power is in knowing what needs to be done.
And having the courage to go out and do it."
Source Unknown

On May 29, 2006 I spent the night in intensive care and faced death again. However, this time it was different, as I chose to be there. I requested the medical profession as my witness that my life living in fear was finally over. This was my day to prove that miracles can happen every day.

"It is time Michelle," were the gentle words spoken by my doctor as I lay in a bed in the Intensive Care Unit (ICU) at the Prince of Wales Hospital, Sydney. With my body in paralysis, I grappled to respond through the almost unbearable taste of fear that was now engulfing my lips. The sound from the heart monitor illustrated the sheer terror going through my veins. The beats accelerated at an expeditious rate.

If I did not cease to exist from being consumed by overwhelming emotions at that moment, I would certainly drown in the sweat. It was now escaping through every pore in my body. It was my moment to leave this world.

What was happening? Why was today so extraordinary? After all, these hospital surroundings were very familiar to me. They were almost like a second home due to the frequency of visits throughout my life.

My "private taxi" as I jokingly called it, came with flashing lights, sirens, and adrenaline. It always had the fastest route to where I had to be in a hurry. I was an adrenaline junky of a different kind who never left home without my EpiPen® (adrenaline auto-injector). I always felt naked and incomplete without it. It was my security blanket. After all, it had saved my life so many times. Ultimately, in an emergency, it was comforting to know that with the adrenaline in my body, I had another twenty minutes to live. Twenty minutes often felt like a lifetime.

My doctor and the intensive care nurses stood around in anticipation with the adrenaline fix armed and ready. They were there to observe what was to happen next—witnesses to a very special farewell to the life I knew so well. It would be my last visit to hospital in this world. And there was no turning back once I stepped into the unknown. As simple as it sounds, I was facing my ultimate demon, which came in the form of a pod or the enclosed edible seed of the plant, Arachis hypogaea. From the legume family, it was best known as a "peanut".

For a brief moment, time stood still and the only sound I could hear was the verbal fusillade inside my head:

I have to do this for myself and others.

Don't worry, it will be okay.

Shit, what am I doing?

Am I crazy?

Oh, my God! Am I really going to eat the peanuts that my doctor is holding in the six jars before me?

Quiet! Quiet!

I must stop this babbling and concentrate,

Oh, shit, I'm scared.

We all have fears and this was my moment to face the biggest one of my life. It was that or continue to hang onto what clearly was not working for me.

What are you afraid of?

In society today, fear comes in many forms. Some people fear public speaking, a new relationship, aging, dying, your first job, illness, saying no, change, being alone, goodbyes, failure, success—the list goes on and on.

For me, I was afraid of living up to my true potential. Today I was going to break that cycle.

My moment of truth had arrived, and an unusual sense of calm and relief filled my body. I was in touch with a very powerful part of myself that knew instinctively that it would be okay. The numbness of missing my family on the other side of the world had now subsided and courage took its place. I was ready.

No words were exchanged, yet I felt an unspoken message from my doctor's eyes saying, "Be brave."

I opened the first of six jars and reminded myself to breathe. The initial challenge to eat this deadly food had presented another one: I struggled to fish out tiny particles of peanut from the end of the jar with my long nails.

This new challenge was no surprise.

I had learned in the past that facing fears was like peeling through the layers of an onion. Once you peel away the first layer, you are presented with more layers, more unforeseen challenges related to that fear. This is the nature of being in unknown territory.

At that point, most will let the feelings of fear overwhelm them. They then decide that they can't handle this new challenge and resort back to going back to what they know. The real courage and power shows up when you make the choice to continue and find a new course of action to overcome the new obstacle that you have been presented with.

"In the middle of difficulty lies opportunity," were the words that flashed through my mind. This was a quote from Albert Einstein that I had seen on a bookshelf in my cousin Pauline's home. After all, touching or smelling peanuts in the past had sent me on a downward spiral.

I picked up a jug of water beside me and created a potentially poisonous cocktail. This was my solution to avoid the touch. Upon drinking this putrid smelly substance, there was no turning back.

If I had an allergic reaction, I would be more focused on what might go wrong. I chose rather to dwell on the positive thoughts of how this event would change my life forever. It was critical to stay positive and achieve the desired outcome for NOTHING to happen.

We sat and waited, scanning my body for allergy symptoms over the next thirty minutes before my doctor took care of other duties.

"Take the contents of the next five jars every thirty minutes thereafter," were his parting words. Each jar contained different amounts of crushed peanuts, with the last containing 6 mg.

"Good luck. I'll see you in the morning." he said, as he walked through the door, waving goodbye.

I was alone.

Up until now I had believed that I was living on the outer circle. It was ironic that I would be situated in an area on the fringe of the ward for this final farewell. To my left, hung the standard swinging doors that led to the main intensive care ward. In front, there was a small window looking out onto the nurses' station.

My only communication with the outside world came via brief conversations with the nurses who popped their heads in regularly to check on my progress. Mobile phones were forbidden.

Unable to contact my family or friends, spoken words were exclusively shared with strangers who were curious to know why I would eat this potentially deadly food in the first place.

"Because my body is telling me that I am ready," was my reply as I worked my way through each jar, slowly gaining confidence as the fear dwindled away.

"Yuck! Is there any beer in the house?" I asked during the periodic check. "Oops! I'm in the wrong place," I thought, smiling to the nurses as my triumph was sinking in.

Comical that this once forbidden food tasted awful, and I was requesting what I thought would be the perfect accompaniment to wash it down.

The tension that once filtered through the faint smell of hospital bleach intermittently was filled with waves of laughter. A small group had now gathered around.

And to my delight, an earthly angel had also been sent to stand among them. The wish I made on the eve of this awakening had been answered. I quietly thanked the universe for sending a familiar face to hold my hand during this ultimate test of courage.

His name was Michael, an acquaintance of a few years. Coincidently, he worked in the same hospital and popped in to visit me. We had only known each other from the chance encounters during some late night drinking binges in the past when we looked our best and the alcohol in the bloodstream had already sent us to oblivion.

Today it was a different setting. I was hooked up to a drip, heart monitor and oxygen reader. I was without make-up, I had frizzy hair, I smelled of sweat and was high on peanut particles.

I had followed the advice of the admissions nurse to wear comfortable clothing. I sat on the bed, wearing the most unflattering light grey track suit pants with black and white stripes on the sides. My favorite homely lilac socks and a red sleeveless singlet. It was not a good look, but it didn't matter today. The true beauty was on the inside, which was now shining.

Michael had come on his day off to hold my hand.

He left as a witness to a miracle.

27
Meeting Destiny

"We can never obtain peace in the outer world until we make peace with ourselves."
Dalai Lama

I sat in my hospital bed exhausted from the last few hours, and if my audience were to return to the room once again, the darkest pair of sunglasses would only offer minimal eye protection from the huge grin now painted across my face.

The heart monitor was beating to the melody of the gurgling from a belly full of peanuts. For the first time, I was laughing at the symphony of weird and wonderful sounds coming from every cell of my body, now dancing in a methodical trance to a sweet music within. If the cells could tell me something, I'm sure they would say, "Let's dance together and embrace this new guest, once dreaded as the ultimate murderous enemy and now welcomed as our friend."

I was distracted by a tapping noise on the doors as they swung open to reveal my cousin Pauline and close friend Craig, beaming with delight. Their presence warmed my heart as they were my only family here, close friend included.

"I can't believe you did it!" Pauline said, swinging a bottle of champagne in one hand and a mysterious bag in the other. "We thought you might like this," she continued resting the brown paper bag beside me. Like a two-year-old, I was curious to discover its mystery, ripping it open to expose all the wonderments inside.

The bag contained a copy of *The Irish Echo*, a newspaper for Irish ex-pats, potato chips, which I ate in my childhood years, a cheddar cheese sandwich—my favorite snack—and lots of other Irish goodies resonating with echoes of home.

"You can save the champagne for later," said Craig, knowing that I'd cherish it as a keepsake of this very special day.

"We can only stay for a short while," Pauline said, glancing at her watch in recognition of the strict ICU visiting time. They were soon to disappear through the doors just as quickly as they had materialized through them. Regardless, I was overjoyed to see two familiar faces, even if only for a brief moment.

The biggest day of my life was nearing a close. Even though I was high, I knew how important it was to catch some sleep to allow this totally new experience to sink into every nook and cranny below the surface of my being.

My eyelids got heavier and heavier, and my head began to sink deeper and deeper into the pillow. It wasn't long before I found myself in a very strange room like that of a futuristic science lab or a painting of minimalist expression. There were no equipment, vials or burners—just open space radiating the essence of everything new and clean. The walls shimmered of metallic silver at first glance, but they were actually transparent, hiding nothing from a heightened sense of knowingness. Lightness filled the air, with no symbols or signs in sight—just the radiance of light emanating from a huge window at one end. The faint hum of a heartbeat was heard through vibrations of love and peace, as if I were in a womb-like state.

"I'm not on my own," I thought, hearing sounds of snoring, deep breathing, and shuffling around. I was surprised to see a sea of crocodiles lying almost motionless on the floor: some were sleeping, others were in silence, and right in the middle of them the biggest and most familiar one of all was staring back at me. But I was calm, unlike encounters before. Freedom was waiting through the opening on the other side.

The only way through was to walk on my tippy toes among them, taking one small step at a time to regulate and maintain a peaceful equilibrium. But just as I got to the opening, the biggest crocodile I had ever seen made a dash for it, landing only inches from my face.

This time he didn't scare me. Instead, I was prepared to stare him down to the finish. Our eyes fixated on each other's, breathing in sync, a mirror image waiting for the first to weaken and crack. As if beams of light radiated from the force of my stare, the space between the spaces dissolved him into particles of specks of dust floating in the air.

Looking for the way out, I felt my way around the window only to discover invisible bars encasing me. The more I noticed them, the more they began to shift and change, gradually becoming opaque to reveal their true form—shape shifters, getting softer and more flexible, the color green transforming into vines.

As if they had minds of their own, they began to wrap themselves around my legs, my arms, tightening my chest to labor my breathing. The sounds of sirens and alarms going off infiltrated this beautiful state. The eerie sound of the heart monitor flatlining rang in my head. Have I reacted? Am I dead?

The dreamlike state dissolved into a bright light.

"Michelle, you are okay. I have you," said an Irish accent in a light-hearted tone

"Where am I?" I thought, dazed and confused that an angel had been sent to me from Ireland.

"You got tangled in all the cords and must have pulled them out of the machines when you turned in the bed," the night nurse said with a smile. "Let me help you detangle yourself," she continued.

"How funny, I thought I had died in my sleep and that you were an angel from heaven," I said to her as I came back to reality. In truth she was an earthly angel, an Irish nurse called Mary who had migrated to Australia only a few months before. I found it uncanny that she came from my hometown and was watching over me on this very special night.

I sat up in the bed, now wide awake. I couldn't help but reminisce about Ireland. Ten years had passed since I first set foot in Australia. I recalled the image of my family imprinted in my mind when they stood at the departure gate as I waved goodbye to them.

"Oh my," A light bulb went on in my head as Dad's words rang in my head as clear as the day he said them: "I believe that we all have a pre-destined path mapped out in our lives. Obviously, yours is guiding you to Australia. And for whatever the reason, one day the light bulb will go on in your head, and you will realize why."

Today I fought the final battle with my enemy and won. I was an ordinary person living the only life I knew, without a doctor's degree, studying art rather than science at school, yet I had overcome what everybody had told me was impossible. It wouldn't have been possible without the people who came into my life for whatever apparent reason. My family was certainly among them, for their unconditional love and support, and for teaching me the most invaluable lesson of all: "No matter how difficult, unforgiving, or impossible challenges seem, the flip side to every problem is that it always has a solution."

The blizzard experience in Washington gave me something to chuckle about. The diagnosis of other health issues came as "blessings"; Andrew came to teach me to take responsibility for my health; many showed up at the right moment, just in time to save my life; John's passing taught me about letting go; Fritz came to guide me towards something I didn't know; muted sound as a child and Luca to show me light I could not see; Craig came to hold my hand in the face of more than one Goliath; my cousin Pauline was there to keep family ties strong, and all the teachers, doctors, and healthcare professionals were there to teach me something I didn't know and to offer a hand of support. The countries I traveled to and every traumatic experience I had encountered each held their own lessons.

I would not be sitting here with a belly full of peanuts if it wasn't for each and every person or experience I encountered—good or bad on my journey—to be here in the present moment. I did not know what lay ahead, but there was a strange familiarity about what I was feeling.

I couldn't help but think of the day I first arrived in Sydney. The bright colors, sounds I had never heard before, the wonderment and curiosity of entering a new unknown world filled with fun and laughter—it all seemed to be bursting at the seams with life.

I placed my head back on the pillow, knowing that my destiny was to bring color, light, fun, and guidance to help others to discover their own destinies. The purpose of my life became clear to me: to light up the room with color *by being* the beautiful essence that I am. I was *to become a teacher, a guide and a shining bright light of inspiration to bring joy into the lives of others through communication, creativity, and love of humanity.*

I wondered what would be my first step in a world without allergies as I drifted off, feeling a sense of inner peace for the very first time.

A Gaelic Blessing...
Deep peace
of the running wave to you,
Deep peace
of the flowing air to you,
Deep peace
of the quiet earth to you,
Deep peace
of the shining stars to you,
Deep peace
of the gentle night to you,
Moon and stars
pour their healing light on you,
Deep peace to you.

This journey is possible for all of us to take. It is a journey that reveals the miracle-working healing power in your own subconscious, an inner world of thought, light, love, beauty, feeling, and power. There are invisible healing forces so mighty that they can open the prison doors of your mind and body and set you free to live your life as the pure flawless diamond you were born to be.

28

My First Step into a New World

"This is one small step for a man, one giant leap for mankind."
Neil Armstrong

There I was, standing in a queue at the checkout of a large supermarket chain in Australia, with chocolate smeared all over my face like a toddler whose birthday had come. I was totally unaware that a crowd of curious shoppers were staring at me like I was some sort of freak. I guess their reaction made sense, given that I was thirty-seven years old at the time.

Why didn't the guy at the checkout call security and have me whisked away in a straight jacket to the nearest loony bin? After all, I was loading a basket full of empty chocolate wrappers onto his conveyor belt, clearly on a rush of endorphins in happy, happy mode. Maybe he didn't have the heart to ruin this euphoric state—or was it just easier to pretend that the "Gobble it up before you purchase" was an everyday occurrence and my behavior was normal?

"Would you like a bag?" he asked, bewildered, as if unsure where to put the pile of rubbish that lay before him. His question somehow caught me by surprise and interrupted this very first delightful chocolate experience.

"Michelle, did they just let you out?" a familiar voice came from the back of the queue. I hadn't noticed my friend Jane amidst the rush of emotions flowing through my body. Nodding to her with acknowledgement and in a fit of giggles, her words only added to the puzzlement of the onlookers, who were probably now wondering, "Let out from where?" and/or "Is she nuts?"...!

It was an acceptable moment of madness, I thought, given the circumstances.

Only yesterday eating chocolate was taboo and potentially life-threatening. A potentially "unsafe food" because of its warning that it "may contain traces of peanuts" normally placed this food in my "no go" zone area. Eating this delight was like playing Russian roulette with my life. There was no way of telling if a bar contained the deadly allergen bullet or not, and therefore eating chocolate had never been a pleasurable experience. I had not known how to live any other way but in survival mode. Today I was teaching myself how to live.

My body was gurgling with delight to a debut rhythm having nothing to compare this first time experience with. I had absolutely no idea of what life held for me, except that my old identity had been wiped clean and there was a whole new world of allergy freedom before me, just waiting to be explored.

Truly, I was an infant in an adult's body—almost like a newborn at birth. Actually, I was. And this new chocolate experience was just one of the many exciting steps on a new adventure exploring unknown territory without Anaphylaxis. Now I could go to restaurants without scrutinizing the menu and interrogating the waiting staff about kitchen practices! I could go to friends' and relatives' homes for dinner without bringing my own food or fear, and without the endless questioning about what they cooked, how they cooked it, and what was on their counters in trace elements. I could order a takeaway when I felt lazy on the weekend.

There would be no more fear of kissing a man who had eaten peanuts in the last twenty-four hours and winding up at death's doorstep! I could give loved ones a huge big hug and never let them go to make up for lost time when they were terrified to get too close. I could pamper myself with cosmetics, have a manicure, get a massage or go to the hairdressers' without worrying about what products they used. I could go back to school or take a trip on a plane without the risk of being singled out as high risk. And, most importantly, I would be able to spend precious moments with my family at peace.

Is it any wonder I was giddy at the possibilities this new world had in store for me?

I couldn't help but think about my perfect fantasy day I wrote in 2003—when I wrote that I would heal my allergies. That was over three years ago, and here I am. It just shows you how powerful the subconscious mind and the body can be when you embrace them.

MY PERFECT FANTASY DAY

I live in a castle surrounded by the ocean and nature. I am a princess of a land filled with nothing but peace and love. It is a world where there is no fighting, trauma or stress, filled with perfect freedom. I feel comfort knowing that my family is close by.

The sun is shining, the sound of the ocean and the air are fresh as all elements of nature rejuvenate my soul.

I am a great painter of color, paving the way for future generations. People travel far and near to see work that touches the hearts of all who gaze upon it. I have embraced powers to communicate with the spiritual world and connect different nations with my visions by use of bright colors and form. I am a great leader for the people, a healer for the sick, and a chosen one to bring some meaning of life to the world.

It is my wedding day. All friends and family from the past and present join together in a peaceful place to rejoice and have fun. They are content and show genuine compassion for each other having put what has gone before them behind. It is a time in the future of peace and brotherly love.

My carriage waits with six white unicorns ready to take me to a clearing in the forest that overlooks a waterfall and a glimpse of the castle in the distance. There I am greeted by my frog – soon to become my prince, powerful by a strong bright eternal light blazing inside for his life long love and devotion to me. Small colorful petals fly through the air, birds sing their songs, and water from the stream nearby trickles past to give life to all.

I found a cure for my allergies, and parents do not have to worry about their children anymore. Today is a feast of nuts and shellfish. There is no fear as we eat in harmony as the day passes.

Teleporting is now possible. Once the ceremony and feast are over, we are transported to another place to share our joy with more family and friends. Everyone is united again, and distance is a thing of the past.

To end the perfect fantasy day, I dance under the moon, free as a bird, accepting the spiritual healing energy from the moon. A star falls from the sky and I make a wish to remain happy forever and to keep love in my heart to be with me tomorrow and always.

Today, I was experiencing freedom for the first time, but most exhilarating was that I had plumbed into the depths of myself and knowledge and I had found answers that had defied medical science.

What is to happen next is crucial to building long-lasting change. There's so much more to tell...

But what I can tell you is that exactly a year later I met my future husband while out celebrating my first birthday with allergy freedom. We were married eighteen months later. Even though we didn't have any unicorns, we did have two wedding ceremonies by the water's edge, both in different locations, two celebrations with friends and family members, and two feasts with peanuts and shellfish.

My perfect day had come true.

29

Leaves from the Pages of Other People's Chapters

"Too often we underestimate the power of a touch, a smile, a kind word, a listening ear, an honest compliment, or the smallest act of caring, all of which have the potential to turn a life around."

Leo F. Buscaglia

I'm including some reflections from others in order to provide some "mirrors" from which my experiences can be seen from perspectives other than my own—to show how Anaphylaxis (acute allergy) impacts not just the life of the person who has it, but everyone who loves and interacts with that person as well.

From my brother:

As a spiritual psychic medium I have learned that through this special gift, our loved ones who have passed to the spirit world can communicate and give messages from the afterlife, therefore allowing healing to take place and to give the sitter the reassurance that we are not ever alone, through whatever circumstance that we deal with in everyday life.

With Michelle there have been times in her life which have really challenged her due to the nut allergy. This led to the feeling of being segregated from doing the same things as her friends, not able to really truly enjoy nights out in restaurants and pubs, etcetera, as we Irish know how to do in style. Even though her feeling different caused grief within that only she could deal with, I know that friends tried to help by being conscious of what they ate in her company, both before meeting her and during. Overall, this had an effect on and placed a burden on some of her friendships, as did enhancing others. This uniqueness beyond her control has led her to be the heart-warming sister she is today.

Her inner knowing that led her to search for something within to help her manage everyday life has opened for Michelle a new chapter. This new birth allows her to enjoy life, releasing the fear that once had caused so much worry and anxiety, to find that special place within, to relax and to find peace.

As a medium, I have realized that sometimes a sitter may come for a reading and just cry, with no words exchanged, but the beauty of healing is that all that is required for the session is a release of emotion. A blockage that a person has carried needs to be released thus, allowing that person to prepare for his or her next lesson in life.

I am very proud of my sister Michelle, and knowing that she will endeavor to help others in anyway possible touches my heart. She will touch many other hearts on her new journey.

Mark Flanagan

From my sister:

Michelle asked me to write a little about how her allergies affected me, her sister. So many thoughts spring to mind!

Living with someone with peanut allergies means you have to be very aware of food. When I get notes home from the school asking parents not to send in any food with nuts, I certainly understand the implications for the children with serious allergies to nuts. The school my children go to post pictures of foods that generally contain nuts, as well as ban children from bringing in cereal bars and some of the other main offenders.

I'm very aware of the extent to which nut traces can be in foods, as going to the supermarket with Michelle used to take hours while she read in detail the ingredients before she purchased. This was also something I had to do when I shared space with Michelle or in latter years when she would visit me. It generally meant that nuts were permanently off my shopping list, as residue from nuts left on surfaces in Michelle's particular case could bring about a reaction. Before she would visit, especially if she was coming for a meal, all kitchen surfaces had to be wiped down.

When we moved to Australia, the allergic episodes for Michelle increased, as did paranoia about attacks—so much so that she would normally bring her own food to parties or try to avoid eating out at all. Sometimes eating out was unavoidable, so in these instances we'd usually have to go to places where they had a "no nut tolerance", which was rare. There were certainly no Thai or Indian takeaways with Michelle back then!

If or when we did venture to a restaurant, which was rare, it was quite uncomfortable for Michelle as she would have to go into detail with the waiting staff about how she had a serious nut allergy and couldn't eat foods with nuts, as well as food that might be prepared near nuts. Sometimes the response from the waiting staff left you wondering if they understood the implications fully, which would leave the rest of us a little uncomfortable as we ate.

All of us in the family and her close friends had to be trained in how to administer adrenaline and the urgency of calling an ambulance. This was always in your mind when you were with Michelle. We knew that knowing this could one day save her life. It was also a similar story when you invited Michelle to someone else's house, but in this case I'd have to explain to the host about her allergy and the precautions they would have to take. This could be a little uncomfortable at times, depending on how well we knew the host. Looking back, when her allergy was at its worst, her social life suffered.

One of the positive outcomes of Michelle's allergy is that she is a great cook, and she hosted many of the dinner parties as that way she was guaranteed she wouldn't serve herself nuts.

Apart from the obvious necessity to be very aware of food around Michelle, I remember being concerned when I was pregnant that my children might have the allergy. So during pregnancy I avoided eating nuts and when my first child was born, I brought her along for allergy tests.

I believe that Michelle's story will go a long way towards educating people about this debilitating allergy. I am proud of her and know that she will do whatever she can to help others affected by this condition and to improve lives if she can.

Paula Flanagan

From my stepmother:

I had no experience of an anaphylactic reaction but through enquiry I realized that this was truly a life-threatening situation. When Michelle was due to come home and live with us for four months in 1998, this really scared and worried me. I cleared out every cupboard in the kitchen and scrubbed them down. I brought Michelle to the supermarket to pick out what hopefully would be safe food for her. Dinner was cooked from scratch every evening, but there was still a fear for me and a huge feeling of responsibility should anything happen to her. Thankfully, nothing did.

In 2006, when we finally received the result that she was now indeed allergy free there was an air of disbelief, delight, and major caution. When Michelle came home a year later minus allergies and we went to a Thai restaurant, I just held my breath and prayed, watching her eat satay sauce. I couldn't believe my eyes when she didn't have any type of allergic reaction whatsoever. It was incredible. I think for a long time I felt great worry and concern for her and needed time to come to terms with this fundamental life transformation, as all the family did. Michelle: Your journey to an allergy free life is incredible and truly inspirational. You, through study, journaling, searching, meditation, and listening to your body have succeeded in releasing yourself from the rollercoaster prison that was your day-to-day life for such a long time.

It is wonderful now when we meet to know you are safe when visiting home, restaurants, and food stores. The freedom of knowing there is no longer the worry of an invisible allergen putting you at risk is such a release from our fear for you.

I believe that your story will educate all who read it to the enormous life limitations for those living with debilitating allergies. It will now give great hope to all who suffer these reactions, their families, friends and colleagues.

Brenda Flanagan

From a friend:

I knew very little about food allergies until I met Michelle at work, and then when we started dating. By talking and getting to know one another, I learned more and more about Michelle's life abroad and her nut allergy, Anaphylaxis. I can still remember our first kiss after I asked Michelle a series of questions: What about your allergy? Do you think it is safe? What about...? She assured me that a kiss would be fine; that she had been quietly watching what I had been eating and drinking all night.

As our relationship developed we went from dating, to moving in together, to working at home together, and to traveling from Australia to Europe. All the while we encountered hurdles and challenges directly related to Michelle's food allergy. On a daily basis there would be challenges like remembering what I had eaten before I would kiss Michelle. This involved knowing the ingredients to absolutely everything I put in my mouth. But I didn't mind because this was something I had to do to keep her safe. Supermarket shopping would always clear the schedule as we had to read ALL the ingredients to EVERYTHING that went into the shopping trolley. This could take up to two hours to complete on some occasions. It just wasn't worth the risk by not checking. Luckily I have always enjoyed supermarket shopping which we turned into a bit of an adventure, and Michelle is a great cook (she had to be).

Holidays would entail knowing exactly where the nearest hospital was. Also, that we stayed in self-catering accommodation so that we could cook our own meals rather than dine out. I was briefed on how to assemble a syringe and administer adrenaline (the days before the EpiPen®), and I witnessed more medical incidents than I would like. I can still remember the panic and helplessness I felt rushing her to the nearest Emergency Room.

Seeing Michelle meet and overcome these challenges on a daily basis, and in many different situations, reinforced my affection and respect for Michelle. The journey she has traversed has been a long and very treacherous one but she has overcome this 'impossible' challenge on her path. I am proud to say that although we are no longer together, I still call Michelle a dear friend.

Craig Ryan

From a friend:

I was chasing the Dream. Getting married, house, kids, secure job, setting myself up for retirement, nice car, holidays, but I was never really happy and content. I had my own awakening at the age of thirty-two in Sydney, Australia, when I got involved with spiritual/holistic healing, personal development, and meditation. I found that these things really worked for me.

When I met Michelle in 1997, I had a few years of personal development under my belt. That is when I upset her asking the "right questions". Why did you create this allergy? What is the advantage for you having this? What are you getting out of it? They are the same questions I ask myself every time a problem or situation is before me. Try it yourself!!!

I have had my fair share of ups and downs in my life. Maybe I will write a book about it some day, but this is about Michelle. Initially, after she was pissed off with me, she began her journey of self-discovery and healing.

The best part is that we have remained friends to this day. I am happy to say that witnessing her journey has helped me immensely in my own life. Michelle has taught me through her own struggle to have a different approach to people with illnesses or any other kind of challenges.

I am more at ease with life, happy and content with the little things, less ignorant and willing to admit my mistakes and apologize when I have judged others. But the most important thing is that Michelle has shown me that anything is possible—that when you take your own journey of discovery, what seems to be the most impossible dream can be turned into reality.

Your body and soul talk to you everyday
So you better listen!

Fritz Jacobi

From a Professional:

Michelle suffered with lifelong debilitating food allergies, and in 2005 found several medical and mind-body therapies to facilitate her return to wellness.

It is important to remember that at the time, a full recovery from food allergy was unheard of.

One of the therapies she chose was Physiotherapy with focus on Ortho-Bionomy®. Ortho-Bionomy® is a gentle form of body work that facilitates the body's own natural ability to return to an improved healthy state.

Michelle at the time was suffering not just from food allergy, but pre-cancerous cells, Grave's disease (a thyroid imbalance), depression, and chronic knee pain and stiffness.

Michelle came to see me for physiotherapy treatment for her chronic knee pain and movement restriction. I have been a physiotherapist all my working life, and in my quest to help people with chronic pain back to wellness, I discovered the highly effective Ortho-Bionomy® modality, which offers most profound transformations to so many of my patients.

With Ortho-Bionomy® we observe that the body in pain will constrict, and with chronic restriction will experience physical symptoms such as pain and stiffness.

Ortho-Bionomy® with its gentle and comfortable hands-on holding of the body, introduces the constricted body to a relaxed state, and very quickly this allows return of movement back to the body's original state, regardless of how long the tension has been there.

As the body experiences comfort, it finds this desirable and seeks to create more, leading the body away from tension and towards healing. This facilitates normal body function and balance, which Michelle found. I know that Michelle first and foremost believed she could heal and had the desire to heal, then took action towards treatments that attracted her, and I observed her progress, moving forward step by small step in her journey towards wellness.

You too can do as Michelle has.

Suzanne O' Hazy
Physiotherapist

From a Professional:

Over the years I have counseled youth at a mental health facility and also acted as a foster parent. I understand the psychological impacts that can result from abnormal environments and traumatic influences. The only exposure I had to allergies was swelling at the site of a bee sting.

After hearing Michelle's story, I was shocked by the severe consequences of those suffering from acute allergic reaction and the events they are forced to experience.

What amazed me more is the dedication and effort Michelle has applied in order to minimize and even resolve her own life-threatening peanut allergy.

My first impression of Michelle was that of an intelligent, carefree, warm, and caring person. We have much in common and often got together discussing world events, our travel adventures, family and well being—all the while laughing at the trials and tribulations of life. As the layers of her personality unfolded, I found her to be a courageous woman of strength and conscientiousness unlike anyone I knew.

The scientific medical field had tainted my belief that mind-body healing was about on the level of voodoo, and some of our conversations left me with my eyes glazed over in polite listening. But the more I did listen, the more I found Michelle had combined a spiritual and professional approach to her accomplishments by furthering her knowledge with accredited education and research regarding the correlation of organ function and the physiological and psychological function of the brain. She has diligently examined areas of cause and effect to the disruption of the complicated workings of the human body and, at the risk of her own life, verified her research.

Irish wit and humor draw you into her journey of inconvenience, loneliness, desperation, fear, and finally to the hope and success of eliminating the threat of an Anaphylactic episode. And her information can be applied to other dysfunctional attributes of the immune system of the human form. Michelle's story approaches many areas of living life with allergies. Unlike the common medical approach to allergy, her experience is definitely a beneficial, if not a life-saving, read for anyone, with or without allergies.

Karon Towns
Journalist & Retired Youth Alcohol and Drug Abuse Counselor

From an Editor:

Working with Michelle as an editor for her book, I became quite absorbed in her journey. I believe that the human being is a marvelous wonder, full of powers we are barely even aware of. Step by step, I followed Michelle into her consciousness and her healing and her communication with her body, retraining it to respond differently to the stimuli that used to bring her close to death. I was fascinated by the idea of retraining the self, even on the cellular level, to unlearn old fears and disable alarm systems that over-react to harmless stimuli. Michelle is a warm, caring human being. She approached all this with great intelligence and tremendous effort, which she modestly attributes to the situation being so grave. She had to delve into her consciousness, which for most of us is a journey that requires great courage.

How many of us avoid looking inside? Sometimes it is for fear of what we will find, sometimes it is sheer laziness (it's a lot easier to turn on the TV!) and some of us find no particular need. Yet, within all of us there is so much truth and power. Through spiritual practices such as Michelle depicts in her book, we can get in touch with our better, more powerful selves, telling ourselves the truth and getting to the level of love. I believe her honesty and bravery can inspire many. She has certainly inspired me with her dauntless courage in the face of "the impossible".

June Saunders

ACKNOWLEDGMENTS

While writing this book, I have encountered the most extraordinary levels of kindness and love. I would like to extend my sincerest appreciation and gratitude to the many individuals for their contributions in helping to turn this book and dream into a reality.

To my immediate family for their relentless support throughout the years, who have lived through everything written in this book and more. Without your love and encouragement, some of my life achievements would still be dreams. My deepest love goes to you.

To my dearest husband, Ennio, who has made so many sacrifices over the years in order to make this book happen. You have been more than patient while putting all of this together. Having you by my side has made all the difference. Your heart knows no limits. *Te amo.*

To my editor June Saunders for your caring and encouragement every step of the way while writing this book. No words can express my sincerest gratitude and appreciation for your input.

To Karon Towns, you not only have made me laugh, but your enthusiam and gift with words is surpassed only by your big heart and hand of friendship. I am truly grateful for everything you have done for me, especially your contribution in this book. I am blessed to have you in my life.

To Laura Bella, you have contributed more ways than you can ever imagine in the shaping of this book. You have been a special friend throughout.

To Ann Harth for your mentoring in the writing of this book, your words of wisdom, and believing in me from early on. Also the same to Jeff Apter and Geoff Bartlett.

A special thanks goes to Fritz Jacobi for speaking the truth, holding my hand on my journey, and for your contribution to the shaping of this book. Also to my dear friends Craig Ryan and Ryan Mcfadden.

To Michelle Keyssecker, Jamie Taylor, Tom Weiner and Alicia Ferris for your support. You took a chance when you didn't have to. I wouldn't have made it this far if it wasn't for you. Thank you!

To Suzanne O' Hazy and Dr. Ulrick for sharing your wisdom, words of encouragement, and for being a good listener. You supported me when I needed it the most.

To Wendy Croxford for your caring and words of encouragement, especially when the end was nowhere in sight.

To Geoff Kabealo for the huge difference that you and your support team have made not only to my life, but to the lives of many. Your personal development courses before PeopleKnowHow ceased were truly a 'turning point' in my life. I am sincerely grateful from the bottom of my heart. "Twinkles"

To Patrick Lemoine, Heidi Goldemund, Sylvie Nobis, Claudia Billenstein, Ciaran Quinn, Aisling Friels, Pauline Dunn, Caroline Cockburn, Paul Farrell, Joe Wrightman, Marcella O'Shea, Marcel Kuska, Jackie Fletcher, Bettina Campbell, Linda Paull, Amy Shakeshaft, Sharon Byrne, Alf Hall, Amy Lawrance, Jodie Skinner, Erika Ballance, Karen Walsh, Jackie Johnston, John Bravar and Bernadette Heathwood; you have seen me at my worst, supported me in some way or another, taught me about courage and bravery, and/or saved my life. I am truly grateful.

To Harold Abrahams, Chris Blackman, Michael Goodman and Terry Ringland, for going out of your way to offer your advice and expertise in your particular fields when you didn't have to.

With special thanks to Nick Cownie from Success Dynamics Institute, and Dennis Hodges N.D. from Naturopathic Services for your contribution. Due to the length of this book, your wisdom is available at www.reactionhq.com.au.

Reaction!
Health Intelligence (HQ)

Appendix: Making Sense

Please note that the information listed in this section of the book is for educational purposes only and must not be used as a substitute or replacement for any advice or diagnosis given by your doctor or health care practitioner.

Appendix: Making Sense
The Battle Just Under the Nose
"Signs and symptoms may reveal a reaction but a reaction cannot come into existence without cause."
Journal Extract: Michelle Flanagan

Below are some snippets from my extensive research on 'hidden ingredients', not just found in food. This section can be used as a reference or guide while reading this book, or simply as a means to increase your Reaction Health Intelligence HQ®.

What Is a Reaction?
Your body is designed to react every second of every day according to the information that it receives and how that information is processed. How you react to this information is determined by how your body has learned to respond to any triggers present. A trigger could be as simple as seeing a photo of a loved one, smelling that person's perfume, hearing his or her name in conversation, etcetera. Has the mention of someone's name ever made your heart beat faster? That person triggers your mind and body to react in such a way.

Once your body is activated, it will react, whether you are aware of the trigger or not, the majority of which lie on an unconscious level, under the surface. They are often difficult to identify, yet you will respond if the right ingredients are present. The good news is that once you identify your hidden triggers it is possible to ultimately change how you react to them. Unfortunately, many of us only explore them when our body is reacting in an adverse way that may pose a threat to our existence.

As our cells continually regenerate, sometimes a 'mistake' is made due to how the initial information is received through the senses. When hidden triggers create an adverse and often undesirable reaction it can show up in the form of an illness, other physical challenge, or even mutation on a cellular level.

Your whole body ultimately believes that it is protecting and healing you. It is following the best strategy possible as to sustain your survival; however, it is sometimes reacting unknowingly, from misperceived information that has been embedded in the cells somehow. I know from my own personal experience that it is possible to correct this misinformation so that the cells react more appropriately. Raising your health intelligence (HQ) is the key to unlocking unwanted reactions and restoring balance.

From the very moment we are conceived, our cells follow the same law which is to survive. This is inherently instilled in every element of our beings and manifests itself through our everyday actions. Every thought you have had throughout your lifetime can be traced to the requirement of how you conducted yourself in relation to your survival. This goes even as deep as one single living cell in your body on its own mission—whether healthy or not the cell will strive to survive. What is cancer but the multiplication of a misinformed, abnormal cell?

Once activated, your body unconsciously does everything it thinks it needs to do to ensure your survival, even if it is mistaken. In extreme circumstances, all thoughts, motivation and actions carried out by you are inherently based on this most basic instinct of all.

Every breath you take and the choices you make about where you work, live, and play all pivot around this innate instinct to survive. Your mind pushes all the unimportant aspects aside and focuses solely on getting through the situation. Your body feels it needs to pull all its resources together to get you beyond the threat to your survival.

Humans are very adept at adaptation. Whatever our life experience is, if we maintain it long enough, we adapt to it, even when it's uncomfortable. Ben Franklin once said that a person only needs to do something for two weeks consistently for it to become ingrained as a habit. We can form good or bad habits that penetrate to the deepest levels of our being and affect our entire lives.

Most people spend their lives searching for answers externally. They forget that they have all the resources that they need inside of them, and that the answers lie in turning inward. Accessing the inner calm changes how you see the world externally and can even affect the external world around you.

The light we are all born with dims as we grow older. Sometimes we have to go back to the beginning to find the light again. To solve a problem, it is important to understand as much as possible about the problem, and sometimes those roots are in our childhoods.

Paradoxically, while technology has allowed the discovery and treatment of new diseases, it has also contributed to their evolution. Evidence shows that new cases of killer allergies and chronic immune-type illnesses are reaching epidemic proportions.

This warns that an upgrade of "health intelligence" is not only timely but crucial. We need to uncover our reactions to hidden factors in the changing environment, the far-from-natural world we live in. This takes more than medicine.

I hope that by knowing these hidden risk factors and how to take charge of our own health will ultimately propel us towards healing our lives and our world.

Health Intelligence (HQ)

Belief

A belief is what we think about ourselves, our lives, and our world, filters of our reality. It is our truth. Learned at a young age from experiencing the world around us we move through our lives by creating similar experiences to mirror our truth. Perception of what is right or wrong, true or false, good or evil, real or unreal stems from beliefs. This is what can propel us forward through life, limit us, or keep us stuck.

Positive belief

"No matter how difficult or impossible the problem, the flip side always holds the solution."

Negative/Limiting belief

"There is no cure and I can't do anything about it."
"I am stuck with this problem."

Disbelief

Disbelief is the inability or refusal to believe or to accept that something is true or real. It is also a lack of faith in something—not believing. If the information received through our senses is distorted, lost, or misinterpreted, our internal filter of what we believe is right or wrong, true or false, good or evil, real or unreal, can become distorted.

Expanded Awareness

The hunter-gatherers used instinctive intelligence to survive; a heightened sensory acuity with an innate ability to sense people, places, and things when the usual five senses of sight, hearing, smell, touch, or taste weren't enough. This expanded their awareness and programmed them with a remote sensing which transcended the rational way of knowing. It is the ability to glean the environment beyond the immediate surroundings through a heightened state of focus, developed out of the necessity to survive.

Decision/Choice

What is the difference between a decision and a choice?
Decisions are made based on the past—from what has been learned from your own life experience or from someone else's. A *decision* is generally made under duress; it has a high energetic charge or past memories attached to it. This can include time and memory distortions, and negative emotions. Negative emotions can include anger, sadness, fear, hurt, guilt, stress, disappointment, shame, overwhelm, frustration, depression, loneliness, tension, inadequacy, rejection, confusion, insufficiency, or repression. Making a decision based mainly on a negative from a past experience, the emotion can be replaced with another negative—pain is held.

Choices are made based on the future—the pros and cons of the situation are evaluated with the future in mind. A *choice* is generally made without duress as it has aspirations and positive emotions attached to it—pain is released.

Types of EGOIC Defense Mechanisms

Self-Centered (obvious)
Defense strategy to protect egoic identity
I will get what I want or need at your expense and do whatever it takes to persuade you to do what I want even if this means a negative response. I will hurt you to win.

Defense Roles
Military style leader, verbal victimizer, bully, dominator, condemner, intimidate, applause seeker, put others down, arrogant individual, aloof or controller.

Self-Centered (hidden/unknown)
Defense strategy to protect egoic identity
I am afraid that I will not get you to do what I want if I am overt about it. Therefore I believe and make you believe that I am not domineering, controlling or manipulating. I give the impression that I am safe to be around, non-controlling, not a competitive threat, or dangerous.

Defense Roles
Seducer, two-faced, chameleon, sincere or charming deceiver, manipulator in a humble way, self-sacrificing parent.

Other People-Centered (obvious)
Defense strategy to protect egoic identity
I meet your needs no matter what. I fear that if I stop meeting your needs something bad will happen to me and that I will feel guilty for hurting you. Therefore at all costs, I will put your needs first as to protect myself from these fears. It is obvious that I am submissive to your needs.

Defense Roles
Martyr, Authoritarian (submissive), obedient servant, depressive (hidden), and proud load carrier as in "I will carry the burden for you'.

Other People-Centered (hidden/unknown)
Defense strategy to protect egoic identity
I believe that I am free, independent and not other people-centered (non-dependant). I will play a role to maintain this belief.

Defense Roles
The Rebel, The Cynic, Freedom, Independent, Organizer/Controller. Aggressive Challenger, Prestigeous, Idol or Status symbol, and Responsible

Avoidance

Avoidance is a defensive mechanism or submissive response to stay away from an uncomfortable situation, which we perceive as a threat, or which we do not understand. This is a learned response for survival that has been passed down from our ancestors. The response to avoid normally follows an intense, highly-charged situation or traumatic event. Avoidance is a common reaction to trauma. If allergen avoidance is what keeps you alive, then it is important to become aware of other types of avoidance, as these can be changed or resolved to alleviate added stress.

Types of Avoidance

Behavioral avoidance is when a person avoids reminders of a trauma or stressful event by changing their behavior to avoid these reminders.

Conflict avoidance is when a person avoids anger, arguments, or potential conflict. Conflict avoiders will please others no matter what and rarely say "no" just to keep the peace.

Emotional avoidance is when a person avoids thoughts or feelings such that the traumatic or stressful event is suppressed.

Social avoidance is when a person feels extreme anxiety around other people. They may fear being scrutinized or evaluated negatively by other people and thus avoid being around others to avoid the fear.

Exercise avoidance is when a person avoids physical exercise to avoid negative feelings about past experiences to do with exercise or a particular action.

"Don't dwell on it", "Put it behind you", "Let's not go there again", "Stay away the next time", "Laugh it off", "Take a pill", "Let's get drunk and forget about it", "Turn your focus to your work", "Go shopping and pamper yourself", "Take a gamble", "Ignore it", "Break ties", "Run and hide": these are just some of the subliminal messages that we become so accustomed to that teach us to avoid.

Rejection/Social Exclusion

In the animal kingdom belonging to a group is a need to ensure survival. It is not a preference but imperative. Social exclusion can crush self esteem and destroy a sense of belonging because it suggests that you have done something wrong or are defective in some way that others do not accept. If belonging to the group or family is under threat so too is well being and survival. Studies at the University of California in Los Angeles (UCLA) have shown that social stress such as the inability to connect with other people can have a major influence on the brain, which in turn affects the immune system, increasing inflammatory activity.

Even brief episodes of being left out or rejected (whether with strangers of not) can lead to a strong emotional and physical reaction. Rejection is so poignant studies have shown that the brain registers it as physical pain. This response makes evolutionary sense because in the times of early man to be rejected not only affected reproduction, but also survival. Individual hunter-gatherers cast out from the group (or tribe) not only left them out of the basic collaboration of food but also to stand alone to face enemies. This often led to illness or death.

So in an evolutionary sense it doesn't matter how tough or sensitive we are, the brain will always register being left out, rejection, ban, singling out, bullying, blacklisting, and exclusion as physical pain. If left unchecked little events can form as one great rejection or physical pain, which in turn with constant reactivity can manifest into trauma on a cellular level without us even knowing.

> Resolve the little moments of upset as they happen.
> This will prevent a build up of subconscious pain and
> trauma from manifesting on a cellular level.

Early Childhood Development and "Mirrors"

Death, Divorce, Separation or Rejection

Apart from the death of a parent, divorce or separation is probably one of the most frightening events in a child's life. The child literally believes that the situation is real. Even though the parents go through their own issues, the young child believes that the breakup is because of him or her—that it is his or her fault, and because of this, they fear abandonment. A child at fifteen to eighteen months old is at its height of separation anxiety. If separation occurs at this age as opposed to any other, fear is intensified and therefore more detrimental to the body.

Sadness/Grief
Part(s) of the body injured by the emotion of sadness/grief: lungs
Gland(s) in proximity to lungs: thymus (immune system)
Challenging time/most vulnerable: 15 to 18 months old (separation anxiety)
Severe cases of sadness/grief injures: lungs and kidneys
Separation/Rejection
Part(s) of the body injured by separation/rejection: heart and lungs
Gland(s) in proximity to heart and lungs: thymus (immune system) and heart (circulatory system)
Associated gland(s): Kidneys (blood filter)
Challenging time: 15 to 18 months old (separation anxiety), imprint period (0 – 7 years), puberty

Fear of Separation

Fear of separation can trigger a strong need to belong, thus by the time a child reaches their teenage years, when they are venturing out into the world as a young adult, rejection or exclusion can be even more damaging to the system.

Part(s) of the body injured by fear of separation: kidneys and heart
Gland(s) in proximity to lungs/kidneys: heart, thymus (immune system), adrenals, testes and ovaries.
Challenging time: 15 to 18 months old, toilet training, puberty, emotional upheaval

Worry

If a child grows up with worry, they learn to fear or feel insecure. Worry can injure the digestive system; therefore the child may become more sensitive to certain types of food. If a child is constantly fed "junk food" that has little or no nutritional value, his or her biological body changes accordingly to accommodate the deficiency. Certain bodily functions fail to perform efficiently; the child may learn bad eating habits, leaving them prone to develop eating and/or digestive disorders later.

Part(s) of the body: Digestive system
Part(s) of the body injured by worry: Digestive system, stomach
Developmental stage: Energetic connections with digestive system form 18 months to 4 years
Other influences: toxins, chemicals, parasites, viruses, certain food processing methods

Fear

A fearful environment may include abuse, violence, fear of monsters or bullies, illness, or watching television, as a child cannot tell the difference between fantasy and reality. Daily fear wears down the sense of security and confidence to move forward in life. The child may become shy when interacting with others, their fear needs attention, yet their environment is unsupported. A worried or traumatized parent or inconsistent boundaries can also trigger fear in a child.

Part(s) of the body injured by the emotion of fear: Kidneys
Gland(s) in proximity to kidneys: adrenal, testes and ovaries.
Challenging time/most vulnerable: toilet training, puberty, stressful situations

Anger

A child who grows up in a hostile environment learns to fight or to hold unexpressed anger. Today, children are exposed to a multitude of images of fighting or violence on TV, fighting with a sibling at home, with a friend at school, and may even witness their parents fight with each other or with others. In this environment a child may feel vulnerable; some toughen up, others learn to stay in "defense mode" ready for conflict; some may become resentful, or may even go out of their way to find trouble. When fear is also active, such as living in a hostile environment combined with the "fear" environment, a child may learn to avoid conflict. They learn that life is a battle; that they must fight or struggle in order to survive.

Part(s) of the body injured by the emotion of anger: Liver
Gland(s) in proximity to Liver: adrenal, testes, and ovaries.
Challenging time/most vulnerable: toilet training, puberty, stressful situations

Shame / Guilt

A child who grows in a shame-filled environment learns to feel guilty. When they are supposed to learn about right or wrong, instead they learn to feel bad about themselves or unworthy. If a parent constantly complains or blames all their wrongdoings on the world or on others, the child can sense this through their heightened sensory acuity and learn to manipulate or control so as to repress the toxic shame subconsciously transferred onto them.

Guilt is the most potent of all emotions and the most negative. It can lead to self-hatred or get us caught in a guilty-about-feeling-guilt loop. We all learn parenting from our parents, they have learned from theirs, and so on. Unintentionally, a parent may deliver the wrong message to the child based on what they learned from their parents. For example, a dad says, 'You are a bad boy.' His child gets the message, 'I'm wrong.' His dad was referring to his behavior, but the child gets the message that he himself is wrong.

Part(s) of the body injured by guilt/shame: Heart
Gland(s) in proximity to heart: heart and thymus (immune system)
Associated gland: kidneys (filter blood)
Challenging time/most vulnerable: toilet training, puberty
Developmental stage: 4 -7 years

Family Systems of Influence

Dominance and Obedience
"I will love you only when you obey."

In this system, Dad is in control, superior and dominant. To win love, you must obey no matter what, it's for the family. Follow the rules, and you will be rewarded. Work hard but don't feel. Home life can be regimented: "Be home at 5pm, or else!" Everything is organized, black or white; Mum is a martyr; good manners are imperative; rituals, religion, and eating can be obsessive; and distrust is high. The coping mechanism is delusion. Perfection, control, power, blame, duty, and martyrism rule. Children in this environment may learn to be competitive for parental affection with other siblings. Therefore, they may have little or no relationship with each other. To live with criticism, a child learns to condemn. A family member may rebel.

Conditional and Unbound
"I love you only when you love me."

In this system, let us all look after each other. "I need your love. I will love you when you love me." There is little or no family structure; there are generally little or no rules as a rebellion against parent's upbringing; therefore any rules put in place may be inconsistent; children are either spoiled or neglected; problems are rarely resolved; parents may act like children, or try hard but never get ahead; and boundaries are blurry. The coping mechanism is denial. Inconsistency reigns: "I will love you if you love me", and the caretaker rule. To live with no boundaries, a child learns to feel unimportant. They may also learn that love is conditional and bring this into their relationships outside of the family system later.

Power and Deception
"I will love you but I have the power to hurt you."

In this system, it is "Let us love each other but lie to each other at the same time". My rights are more important than yours; do what you like—just don't get caught; the environment is abusive; family loyalty is high no matter what; members are shamed to feel or need; the family boundary is rock solid to keep non-family members out; and members have to be tough to survive. The coping mechanism is delusion. Punishment, power, and control rule.

"Mirrors" of Influence on the Energetic Body

"Don't tell your sister", "Speak only when you are spoken to", "Children should be seen and not heard" are just a few of the subliminal messages we pick up during our developing years. In this case, in an energetic sense the body learns to hold back the urge to speak up, to express, or to be heard? Thus tightens an invisible belt around the voice box and surrounding throat area to restrict it, to stop the impulse or flow of energy to that part of the body. The consequences of speaking up when told not to creates fear in the child. Fear that if the belt is loosened, trouble waits around the corner.

Our ancient ancestors believed that our bodies develop an energetic blueprint in early childhood, one that can stay with us through adulthood unless we become aware of it. Whatever the message, if repeated over a long period of time, our unique energetic blueprint is imprinted into the body's internal guidebook.

Evidence shows that our bodies produce a complex network of chemicals (neuro-transmitters, neuro-peptides, and related molecules) that our brain uses to communicate throughout the body. How these messengers flow around the body can influence emotional, physical, and mental health. If certain parts of the body are energetically blocked or have no boundaries to contain or receive these messengers, then information communicated from the brain to the body may get lost, misinterpreted or misunderstood.

What we learn as children is determined by our age, stage of physical, mental, emotional development, surroundings, intense events and/or a lot of little things of which you don't yet understand. These developmental sequences or markers, mostly the same in all children, are linked to the maturing of the central nervous system.

By the time we reach adulthood the initial physical sensations that once created the energetic habits are consciously forgotten. But the subconscious remembers. So much so, that it waits until the right ingredients are present in the internal or external environment to trigger the sequence of actions and reactions initially learned.

Humiliation, neglect, rejection, doubt, anger and jealousy are just some of the many ingredients that can trigger the sequence or physical response. Most of which occurs on a subconscious level, unaware that our body and mind has physically reacted. This means that unknown to us, unresolved feelings such as jealousy from a past environment, if present in current surroundings, could trigger an energetic surge under the surface. For example, you may believe that you are not a jealous person but on a subconscious level, the energy of this emotion may wait for the right ingredients to activate. Simply by becoming aware of increased activity in your body at certain times or when unwanted situations just seem to repeat over and over again—this may indicate an unresolved emotion.

Energetic ties or habits can harm the body on a deeper level if their ingredients or triggers are left unresolved. It is important to recognize your energetic habits to identify what can harm or heal your life, to become aware of hidden triggers, and to take the time to resolve them.

Bioenergetic Exercise

Bioenergetic exercise has been likened to "yoga with sound" — with additional expressive motions. Bioenergetic exercises allow for an emotional release through laughing, shaking, and/or positioning the body in a certain way to release unconscious negative emotions held deep in the body. This type of exercise can be performed by both children and adults. An example of bioenergetic exercise is outlined in Chapter 20: The Sound of Silence; the exercise involves releasing tension surrounding the throat area.

The Nervous System

When starting out on my path of healing I believed it important to know how to distinguish the difference between the fighter and the peacekeeper. This directed me to learn about the human nervous system, the system responsible for the "fight or flight" response and other reactions. It also led me to look at 'hidden ingredients' with fresh eyes.

The human nervous system has two main divisions: the central nervous system and the *autonomic* nervous system.

The *central nervous system* is the conscious part of the system, the brain and spinal cord concerned with sensory input received through the senses, integration of data, and motor output.

The *autonomic nervous system* is the subconscious part of the system which we have less conscious control over. These include the digestion of food, blood pressure, breathing, and heart rate. The nerves extend from the spine connecting to organs and glands that stimulate or suppress their function. The subconscious part has two branches: the *sympathetic nervous system* that activates glands and organs to defend the body against attack, and the *parasympathetic nervous system*, which is concerned with rebuilding the body through nourishment, elimination of waste, healing, and cell regeneration.

The Sympathetic Branch of the Nervous System

The *sympathetic* branch is primarily aroused in states of extreme stress (both positive and negative), trauma, a build up of stress over time, a threat, blue light (covered later), and intense emotional states such as rage, desperation, fear, terror, anxiety, panic, and trauma, which provoke the body's readiness for fight or flight.

A small part of the brain called the amygdala, an internal survival mechanism since prehistoric times, alerts of danger or a perceived threat in the surroundings. It works faster than the thinking part of our brain and responds instantaneously. It is important for survival as it prepares our body to fight the danger or flee from it.

Under normal circumstances, both systems function in balance with each other to maintain metabolic equilibrium. When one side is up, the other side is down; they swing in complementary balance. However, in extreme circumstances, when the fight/flight response is not possible, such as when there is no time, strength or stamina to succeed, the nervous system commands the body to freeze; to go into paralysis. This can be seen in nature when animals such as a mouse in the mouth of a cat may "go dead". Its muscles lose tone, and the body is limp like a rag doll. This is when the *sympathetic* remains activated but the *parasympathetic* simultaneously becomes highly activated, thus masking the *sympathetic* activity and causing the body to go limp.

The Parasympathetic Branch of the Nervous System

The *parasympathetic* branch is primarily aroused in states of rest, relaxation, sleep, pleasure, sexual arousal, and emotional states including happiness, grief, and sadness. This system maintains balance, fine-tuning organs in relation to each other so as to keep up with the demands of the internal maintenance, shift, and change. This system may activate or suppress functions of one organ or body part, or it may affect global systems—for example, turning off the whole skeletal musculature during dream sleep. It promotes rebuilding, cell growth, and conservation of energy.

Noticeable signs of the *parasympathetic* branch include slower, deeper respiration and heart rate (pulse), pupils constrict (get smaller), salivation increases, muscles relax, digestion increases, skin is flushed, and the person may retreat into mental, internal life.

The Fighter Versus the Peacekeeper

Both systems have very distinct roles: one is to defend and protect, and the other is to maintain, restore, and heal. Physical symptoms such as a cough or sneeze happen after an initial threat has been detected. These types of reactions are effective ways to remove unwanted debris or foreign particles from the lungs or respiratory tract.

Vomiting, which I call a stomach sneeze, expels harmful substances from the stomach and small intestine. Diarrhea is a quick response to remove harmful substances that may be irritating the intestines. Swelling or inflammation prevents the invader from entering the bloodstream, mobilizing it for combat.

These acts of expulsion restore balance rather than attack or defend. I believe this is why people sometimes confuse the immune system with the healing system. Both systems work in a cooperative effort to maintain survival. Both systems adhere to the most basic instincts and needs of human survival—food, water, air, shelter, and sleep. For example, if the body is low on energy, the healing system prompts eating; whereas the immune system attacks viruses, toxins, bacteria, or other contaminants found in the food.

If water reserves in the body are low, the healing system tells us to drink to prevent dehydration. The immune system then defends against parasites or contaminants found in the water. If shelter is too hot or too cold, then sweating or shivering may occur. This serves to cool or heat the body and to trigger another response such as to take off or put on a coat. If the body is under attack by a virus, it turns up the heat to create unfavorable conditions for the virus to exist. Heat serves as a defense mechanism and assists the healing system. If the *parasympathetic* branch is overactive, then this may result in an underactive thyroid gland (hypothyroid). If the *sympathetic* nervous system is underactive, the adrenal or pituitary glands may become underactive (hypo).

Symptoms of the Fight/Flight Response

During the "fight" or "flight" response, chemicals are released into the bloodstream to respond to the perceived threat. Pupils dilate, heart and breathing rate increase, muscles tense, skin pales, there are tremors or shivering or sweating; goosebumps may appear on the skin, digestion slows down, sexual arousal is halted, the sense of smell is heightened, salivation in the mouth decreases, and concentration focuses on the specific. Its principal function is the control of short range, moment by moment adaptation. Activation shunts the body away from metabolic energy and long-range developmental activities.

Prolonged Reactivity of Fight or Flight

Even after the fight/flight response is long over, the resistance reaction allows the body to continue fighting the stressors long after the effects of the alarm system have dwindled. It is a vicious cycle, first set in motion by survival, but enduring as impairment. When the state of emergency or trauma is unresolved over long periods of time, the body reserves become depleted and the immune system weakens. Constant fight/flight reactivity can cause muscle tension and lead to zinc, magnesium, sodium, copper and calcium imbalances. (See more on page 299 and from page 317)

Prolonged reactivity over a long period of time may lead to fatigue, shock, adrenal exhaustion, kidney imbalance, hyperthyroidism, bodily damage, nervousness, and scanty perspiration. The situation may then skew normal cognitive and cell regeneration function, severely impair the ability of the immune system to function, and, in extreme cases, the system may collapse or lead to death.

When *sympathetic* arousal is constantly high, adding a new stress shoots it up even higher, causing the feeling of being overwhelmed. Anxiety, irritability, and nervousness are common, including having more active or overactive thyroid and adrenal glands, as these are activated by the *sympathetic* nervous system.

The Biochemical Stress Response

The hypothalamus in the brain releases the hormone corticotrophin-releasing hormone (CRH). This travels to the pituitary gland to trigger the release of adrenocorticotropic hormone (ACTH). This hormone instructs the adrenal glands to release a third hormone, cortisol, known as the stress hormone. The adrenal glands, located above the kidneys, produce three kinds of steroid hormones which include mineralocorticoids (aldosterone), glucocorticoids (cortisol), and small amounts of sex hormones.

Aldosterone

Stimulated by the pituitary gland, Aldosterone, a mineralocorticoid, is secreted from the adrenal glands to tell the kidneys to retain more sodium and copper and to eliminate large amounts of zinc and magnesium. During the fight/flight response, magnesium in the muscles is removed and replaced with calcium from the bones.

Calcium gives the muscles their rigidity in preparation to fight or flee. Once the stress is over, the magnesium rarely re-enters the muscle cells again, as it has been eliminated. Zinc and magnesium are calming minerals which complement the *parasympathetic* branch, so if levels decline due to constant "fight or flight" activation, the ability to cope under stress is greatly impaired.

The Stress Hormone: Cortisol

In our modern world we cope with stress all the time: in the workplace, at home, from chemical and toxin exposure, excessive caffeine, waiting in line, etcetera. Under chronic stress secretion of the stress hormone, cortisol is secreted most of the time. Constant secretion can damage the body. Cortisol, produced in the adrenal glands, is a glucocorticoids that raises the level of glucose in the blood by stimulating the liver to release stored sources into the blood, making more energy available to fight or flee. It also inhibits the immune system in order to reduce inflammation. Following an acute allergic reaction, *prednisone,* derived from cortisol, is used to treat swelling. Elevated levels of cortisol are specifically toxic to brain cells, interfering with the production of new brain cells, and this can adversely affect memory and thinking. Cortisol activity is intertwined with insulin and blood sugar levels, which can lead to the risk of diabetes and an increase in abdominal fat.

Chronic Stress

It would make perfect sense that if the *sympathetic* branch is frequently activated, then *tyrosine* would surely signal the synthesis of an excess of epinephrine. Studies have shown that chronic stress may lead to the production of certain immune factors called cytokines which can produce a damaging inflammatory response. Cortisol inhibits the immune system to reduce inflammation. Therefore, high levels of cortisol can affect immune function. An accumulation of belly fat is a sign of abnormal blood sugar and insulin levels.

As blood flow to the skin during a stress response is reduced, chronic stress can lead to skin conditions such as acne or rosacea (facial reddening) as the healing system's effort to send blood to areas starved of essential nutrients. Some evidence suggests that repeated release of stress hormone produces hyperactivity in the hypothalamus-pituitary-adrenal axis and disrupts normal levels of serotonin.

Adrenal Weakness

Symptoms of adrenal weakness or exhaustion may include chronic fatigue, depression, anxiety, infections, lower back pain, problems with weight, anger, hypoglycemia, inability to focus, poor memory, fibromyalgia, thyroid problems, sweet cravings, feeling cold, or any chronic or autoimmune disease. It is known that a deficiency of adrenal hormones causes a hypersensitivity to other hormones such as thyroxine (thyroid) and insulin (pancreas).

Some studies suggest that hypoglycemia, a hypersensitivity to sugars can result from an adrenal hormone deficiency, which can be corrected with vitamin B5 (a cortisol precursor).

Epinephrine

Epinephrine (also known as adrenaline), a hormone and neurotransmitter (chemical messenger) is secreted from the adrenal glands in response to stress. Epinephrine is used in the event of an anaphylactic reaction. Epinephrine, derived from the amino acids phenylalanine and tyrosine, moves oxygen-rich blood to the brain and to the muscles required to fight or flee by increasing heart rate, constricting blood vessels, and dilating air passages. Epinephrine causes the release of fatty acids and glucose into the bloodstream to create more energy. Therefore, stress can impair the clearance of fat molecules in the body and temporarily raise blood-cholesterol levels.

The Origin of Epinephrine

Phenylalanine

Phenylalanine is naturally found in breast milk, nature's way of telling us that it as safe for consumption from a very young age. Phenylalanine, in its synthetic form, is used in the manufacture of food and drink products and some nutritional supplements. Phenylalanine and tyrosine compete with tryptophan for absorption.

Tyrosine

Phenylalanine is a precursor for tyrosine, an amino acid used by the cells to synthesize proteins, dopamine, norepinephrine, (noradrenaline), epinephrine (adrenaline), and the skin pigment melanin. Tyrosine gets its name from the Greek, meaning *cheese*, first discovered in 1846 in the protein casein from cheese. It is found in many high protein food products such as peanuts, almonds, fish, soy products, chicken, turkey, avocados, milk, yogurt, cottage cheese, lima beans, pumpkin seeds, and sesame seeds. Most of these foods are known to induce an anaphylactic reaction. Tyrosine and phenylalanine compete with tryptophan for absorption.

Melanin

Hair receives its color from different amounts of melanin pigments found in the outer layer of the hair. Melanin is also responsible for skin color and is affected by sunlight. Melanin is regulated by the endocrine system, in particular the adrenal glands. Deficiency in kidney function and/or adrenal hormones can be indicated by loss of hair coloring or gray/white hair. There is a direct correlation between shock or extreme stress and hair loss or gray hair. Healthy-looking hair essentially requires nourishment from blood flow, held in place and maintained by the *sympathetic* branch of the nervous system.

A lack of nutrition or nervous exhaustion resulting from prolonged stress can literally deliver a bad hair day.

Touch
The Cuddle Hormone: Oxytocin

Oxytocin stimulates the uterine contractions of labor that are needed to move the child out through the birth canal. The hormone stimulates the release of milk from the mammary glands by causing surrounding cells to contract. After birth, stimulation of the breast by the infant feeding stimulates the posterior pituitary to produce this hormone. Oxytocin also plays a role in social interaction and reproduction. Studies show that a hug reduces the level of cortisol (the stress hormone) in the bloodstream.

Touch Anchor

A touch anchor can form in the midst of an intense emotion such as crying or deep upset when another may hug or offer a touch of support on a particular part of the body, such as tapping your shoulder. If this same spot is touched repeatedly over time while this same intense emotional state is activated;, the body learns to link that particular emotion and the sensory sensation together. This creates an unconscious "button" that can be activated at any time simply by repeating the step. This means that every time, in this case, when the particular part of the body is touched the feeling of upset is also ignited.

In society when consoling someone we have learned acceptable places to reach out and touch someone as an instinctive response to offer some comfort. This means that as we go through life we are left with a multitude of subconscious anchors or buttons on the surface of the skin that, once pressed, can release a whole array of unexplained emotions that stem from our pasts and increase in intensity over time. Touch can be anchored to a positive or negative emotion.

The next time you are in the throes of laughter such as by watching your favorite comedy on TV, remember to touch or pinch a particular unique part of your body to create a touch button to link it to that positive emotion. Repeat about three times. You will know that this anchor has been successfully installed when you touch that spot and the emotion fires off in the absence of the original stimulus. Replace touch with a certain food, smell, sound, or image/color to create an alternative sensory anchor to a positive emotion.

The Digestive System and Stress

During stress or fight or flight response, the digestive system is suppressed or slowed down. If stress is prolonged over a long period of time, this can impact digestion and the body's ability to absorb essential nutrients and energy in order to function efficiently. This in turn can lead to damage on a cellular level, disrupt normal sleeping patterns and circadian rhythms, leave the body vulnerable to infection and/or parasite and virus infestation, alter DNA, deplete nutrition and energy levels, suppress immune function, and disrupt innate healing capabilities.

Serotonin

Serotonin is derived from the amino acid tryptophan, 80% of which is located in the gastrointestinal tract, the main digestive highway. Serotonin is a principal regulator of pain, appetite, sleep and mood. Low serotonin levels have been associated with anxiety, irritability, depression, impatience, impulsiveness, weight gain, overeating, inability to concentrate, carbohydrate cravings, insomnia, and poor dream recall.

The Origin of Serotonin

Tryptophan

Tryptophan is one of the ten essential amino acids that the body uses to synthesize protein. It is converted into niacin (vitamin B3) by the liver and is known for its production of nervous system messengers, especially those related to relaxation, restfulness, and sleep, traits of the *parasympathetic* nervous system. It has a powerful calming, anti-anxiety, and anti-depressant effect. Vitamin B6 is necessary for the conversion of tryptophan to niacin and serotonin. Vitamin B3 and C also play a role. Tryptophan located in the upper gastrointestinal tract converts to melatonin during fasting but more so just after food intake. Evidence shows that long term fasting can decrease melatonin secretion from the pineal gland yet increase it in the gastrointestinal tract.

Tryptophan is found in red meat, nuts, seeds, dairy, bananas, soybeans, soy, tuna, shellfish, and turkey. Incidentally, nuts, seeds, dairy, bananas (latex), soybeans, soy, and shellfish are known foods that can trigger an anaphylactic allergic reaction. Tryptophan can also be found in some baby formulas. Tyrosine and phenylalanine compete with tryptophan for absorption.

Trypsin/Chymotrypsin

Trypsin and chymotrypsin are substances secreted for normal digestion. Trypsin and chymotrypsin are structurally very similar, although they recognize different substrates. Trypsin acts on lysine and arginine, and chymotrypsin acts on large amounts of tryptophan, tyrosine and phenylalanine. They are produced in the pancreas. When the pancreas are stimulated, digestive enzymes travel via the pancreatic duct to the small intestines.

Trypsin breaks protein down so that it can be absorbed through the lining of the small intestines. During times of stress and/or the fight or flight response, secretion of digestive enzymes from the pancreas is inhibited; also, sphincters in the small intestines contract to decrease motion and to stop the flow of partly digested food passing from the stomach to the small intestine. When the pancreas does not produce adequate amounts, this can be detected in a stool sample.

Trypsin can be used to break down casein in breast milk. If trypsin is added to a milk powder solution, the breakdown of casein will cause the milk to become clear or translucent. It is used to dissolve blood clots in its microbial form and treat inflammation in its pancreatic form. In the laboratory, biological researchers use trypsin to digest proteins into peptides for mass spectrometry analysis, also sometimes used in vaccines to break up monkey cells and other flesh in vaccine cultures. It is also added to baby food to pre-digest it. This breaks down the protein molecules, which helps the baby to digest, as its stomach is not strong enough to digest bigger protein molecules. Trypsin is destructive to proteins. Is this addition to baby and infant products necessary, especially when nature did not intend for them to have trypsin in abundance when the immune system is still in its infancy?

Lysine

Trypsin breaks down lysine, an essential amino acid which the human body cannot synthesize itself. Therefore, it must be ingested. L-Lysine is a necessary building block for all protein. It plays a major role in absorption of calcium; building muscle protein; production of hormones, antibodies and enzymes; and assisting in recovery after a muscle injury. It can also affect serotonin levels in the gastrointestinal tract. Animal studies suggest that a lysine deficiency can cause immunodeficiency. Lysine is found in foods rich in protein, such as soy, meat, cheese (particularly Parmesan), eggs, cereal grains, and fish (cod and sardines). It is plentiful in most legumes. Studies show that a lysine deficiency can increase serotonin levels in the amygdala, the part of the brain involved in the fight/flight response and emotional regulation. Lysine is used in animal feed as a low cost protein alternative. It is industrially produced by microbial fermentation, from a base mainly composed of sugar.

Arginine

Trypsin also breaks down arginine, an amino acid naturally produced in the body. This plays an important role in cell division, ammonia removal (urea), wound healing, immune function, and it helps to reduce blood pressure and aids in the release of hormones. It is a precursor for the synthesis of nitric oxide. Increased intracellular calcium, in conjunction with excess excitatory amino acids and nitric oxide, has been associated with several neurodegenerative diseases. Arginine (8%) is added to dental products such as toothpaste to provide relief from sensitive teeth. The Mayo Clinic reports that inhalation of L-arginine can increase lung inflammation and aggravate asthma. Arginine can be found in dairy products, pork beef and poultry, gelatin, seafood, wild game, peanuts, nuts, wheat, granola, seeds (pumpkin, sesame, sunflower), soybeans, and chick peas.

The Pineal Gland/Melatonin

Melatonin

Melatonin is made from tryptophan and serotonin; production depends on the same nutrients used in the making of serotonin. This hormone is secreted by the pineal gland to regulate circadian, the daily body clock, and the sleep/wake cycle. It is a serotonin derivative *melatonin* which means "night worker" (it is from the Greek, melos, meaning "black", and tosos, meaning "labor"). It is also known as the "hormone of darkness". This is secreted by the pineal gland mainly in response to darkness in both day-active and nocturnal animals. This hormone, which is sensitive to light, communicates information about environmental lighting to various parts of the body.

Melatonin acts like a powerful antioxidant, in that it protects nuclear and mitochondrial DNA. In the upper portion of the gastrointestinal tract (GIT), studies have shown that melatonin displays a wide variety of activities such as free radical scavenging, circadian entrainment, and it protects the lining of the GIT from irritants in addition to aiding in the healing process in this area when it comes to ulcers, gastritis, esophagitis and stomatitis. "Itis" means inflammation or swelling.

Mitochondrial DNA (mtDNA) *is the DNA of the mitochondrial chromosome, existing in several thousand copies per cell and inherited exclusively from the mother. Mitochondrial are structures within eukaryotic cells (cells with nuclei) that convert the chemical energy from food into a form that cells can use.*
Nuclear DNA (nDNA) *is the DNA of the chromosomes found in the nucleus of a eukaryotic cell and inherited from both parents.*
Source: *Wikipedia* and the *Farlex* online medical dictionary

According to Maestroni (1993), in an article in the *Journal of Pineal Research*, "A tight, physiological link between the pineal gland and the immune system is emerging from a series of experimental studies. Pinealectomy or other experimental methods which inhibit melatonin synthesis and secretion induce a state of immunodepression which is counteracted by melatonin.

It seems important to note that one of the main targets of melatonin is the thymus, i.e., the central organ of the immune system. That melatonin appears to have an immunoenhancing effect."

Melatonin presumably acts like a local hormone in bone cells since it is found in high quantities in bone marrow (not blood borne), where cell precursors (such as immune system mast cells) are located. Melatonin levels can also be seen during the day. Recent studies show melatonin in the upper part of the gastrointestinal tract (the oral cavity such as in saliva, the esophagus, stomach and duodenum) and is released during the day while fasting but much more after food intake. Melatonin released in response to darkness is from the pineal gland, whereas if produced during daylight, it comes from the gastrointestinal tract. Evidence shows that long term fasting can decrease melatonin release from the pineal gland yet increase it in the gastrointestinal tract, whereas pineal production remains unaffected by eating. One of melatonin's main targets is the thymus gland, i.e., the central organ of the immune system.

Studies have shown a link between the tonsils and melatonin, indicating that melatonin plays a role in relieving symptoms of acute tonsillitis. If the presence of melatonin is known to alleviate inflammation of the tonsils, then surely a deficiency could result in acute inflammation in the area, especially when a foreign substance has been ingested or inhaled. If tyrosine and phenylalanine (epinephrine) compete with tryptophan (serotonin) for absorption, then this would surely mean that with digestion slowing down during the fight/flight response, serotonin/melatonin in the gut and bone marrow are inhibited or suppressed. The bone marrow is the place where calcium is stored—the calcium that replaces muscles with magnesium during times of stress. It is also where mast cells associated with the immune response in allergic reactions are produced. With melatonin/serotonin suppresed, nuclear and mitochondrial DNA and protective lining/mucosa are left unprotected.

During stress the mitochondria, the internal power plant of the cell, can bind to a certain amount of calcium. When this calcium builds to a certain point, it can deactivate the mitochondria, thus forcing the cell to increase its energy production, which produces an excess of lactic acid. Dying or stressed cells take up calcium while exciting the cell at the same time. This intensifies stress. A cramp is an example of uncontrolled cellular excitation. Prolonged excitation and stress can lead to tissue inflammation. Cortisol, the stress hormone, can take over to reduce inflammation, thus inhibiting the immune system.

In 1917 cow's pineal extract was found to lighten frog skin. Dermatology professor Aaron B. Lerner and colleagues at Yale University, hoping that a substance from the pineal might be useful in treating skin diseases, isolated and named the hormone melatonin in 1958. During stress, blood flow that brings nutrients and minerals to the skin is suppressed, thus it can create a similar outcome as in the GIT scenario outline above. Prolonged stress can create a build up of acid under the skin, which can lead to skin irritation or inflammation.

Tonsils / Melatonin

Tonsils have a privileged situation in the immune system in that they are in touch with the environment. Studies have shown a link between the tonsils and melatonin indicating that melatonin plays a role in relieving symptoms of acute tonsillitis. That if the presence of melatonin is known to alleviate inflammation of the tonsils then surely a lack of it could result in acute inflammation in the area when a foreign substance has been ingested or inhaled.

24 hour cycle - Peak energy/activity of organs		
Most Active	**Organ** (Peak Energy Flow)	**Mental/Emotion** (weaken/injure area)
7-9 a.m.	Stomach	Worry, fear, and intimidation
9-11a.m.	Spleen	Sensitivity to criticism
11a.m.-1p.m	Heart	Hate, greed, insecurity
1-3p.m.	Small Intestine	Cruelty, hate, impatience, indiscretion and impatience. Injury can lower self-esteem, self-respect, and confidence
3-5p.m.	Urinary Bladder	Fear, suspicion, jealousy
5-7p.m.	Kidney	Prolonged fear
7-9p.m.	Circulation/Sex Protects the heart	Sadness, emotional stress, and external heat or pressure
9-11p.m.	Abdomen, Chest and Pelvis	Distrust, lack of creativity, emotional upset, break up or separation, suspicion
11p.m.-1a.m	Gallbladder	Anger, frustration, resentment, lack of control, bitterness
1-3a.m.	Liver	Discontent, anger, and frustration
3-5a.m.	Lungs	Sadness
5-7a.m.	Large Intestines	Money and sex

Light
The Electromagnetic Spectrum

The Electromagnetic Spectrum consists of radio waves, microwaves, infrared radiation, visible light, ultraviolet rays, x rays, and gamma rays. Visible light (the visible part of the electromagnetic spectrum) comprises all those electromagnetic radiations that the human eye can detect such as color.

Photons

Prior to Einstein little was understood about light. The term 'photon' was born out of his theory which focused on electron emissions and energy transfers. Basically light is made of photons which are individual packets of energy. A photon lacks mass but has both an electric and a magnetic component (wave and particle duality) and travels from the sun at the speed of light. Each photon has a difference between them, not by its speed but by how it moves.

Every single photon moves forward in a zigzag or wave-like motion traveling at exactly the same time, at approximately 300,000 km/sec. They change shape, mutate, or do something different depending on their wave-like motion which can be described in one of three ways: by wave frequency (hertz), wavelength (meter), or by energy (eV).

The frequency of a wave is determined by the number of complete waves, or wavelengths, that pass a given point each second for example one wave (or cycle) per second is 1 Hz. The distance measured between each crest is the wavelength. Therefore longer waves have less wave frequency and lower energy/intensity of photons, energy which is measured in units of electron volts (eV).

Radio Waves

At one end of the spectrum are the longest wavelengths called *radio waves*. They can be as long as the planet or as short as a football which can transmit music, conversations, pictures and data invisibly through the air, often over millions of miles.

Microwaves

The next on the spectrum are *Microwaves* that can heat food by forcing fat and water molecules in food to rotate thus cooking the food. These waves can penetrate through clouds, rain, snow, and smoke, often used in weather forecasting systems, radars, in telecommunications and broadcasting and satellite communications systems. Both radio and microwaves are measured by frequency (Hz).

Infrared Radiation

Then there's *infrared* radiation (measured by wavelength) which when interacting with matter can set molecules to vibrate thus creating heat. We can see infrared radiation as heat (thermal) using 'night vision' goggles and certain animals and reptiles like snakes can sense infrared thermal radiation which allows them to find prey in the dark.

Visible Light

Our atmosphere is literally full of photons traveling at different frequencies yet humans are only able to see a very small fraction of them. Visible light is a narrow band roughly in the middle of the spectrum. These photons zigzag once between approximately 400 (violet end) and about 700 nanometers (red end) with blue, cyan, green, yellow and orange in between.

Violet – Indigo – Blue – Green – Yellow – Orange – Red
400 nm   500nm   600nm   700 nm

A nanometer (nm) is one-billionth of a meter

Shorter Wavelengths	Longer Wavelengths
Higher Frequency	Lower Frequency
Higher Photon Energy	Lower Photon Energy
Electric/Magnetic Energy	Thermal Energy

As wavelengths contract or get shorter towards the blue/violet end of the spectrum, the frequency and photon energy increases. This means that *red* light has longer wavelengths, less frequency of waves, and lower photon energy/intensity than *blue* light.

White Light

When all the visible wavelengths are present in equal amounts *white* light or nearly *white* light from the sun is perceived. Technically *white* is not a color but rather a continuous distribution of wavelengths.

Ultraviolet Light

Beyond the visible spectrum is *ultraviolet* (UV) light which you cannot see. The sun is a strong source of ultraviolet radiation, but atmospheric absorption such as air eliminates most of the shorter wavelengths. UV light can make things glow or become florescent, experienced as sunburn when near *ultraviolet* is absorbed in the surface layer of the skin. A bumble bee can see ultraviolet light.

X-Ray

The next below UV on the spectrum are called *X-rays* also invisible to the naked eye but allows us to see bones.

Gamma Rays

Then, finally *gamma rays* which have the shortest wavelength on the other end of the spectrum generated by radioactive atoms and in nuclear explosions. This frequency has deadly super-high energy which can smash and kill cells, lead to mutation and destroy DNA.

The Effects of Visible Light on the Body

Some visible light frequencies from the electromagnetic spectrum and their influence on the body

Red

Red is at the lowest end of the visible light spectrum, and has a frequency range of 700nm (longer wavelengths, lower energy, lower frequency). Red relates to the base of the spine, kidneys, bladder, hips, legs and the adrenal glands. Red stimulates and strengthens physical energy and is therefore helpful for tiredness and lethargy. However, a red light placed beside the bed at bedtime can stimulate the *parasympathetic* nervous system. Red can also be used to raise the body's temperature and to help boost sluggish circulation by energizing blood flow. High blood pressure can indicate too much red energy within the body. When the air is polluted with small particles a sunset will be red.

Positive aspects of this frequency:
Energetic, leadership, strong willed, spontaneous, determined, pioneering, confident, and courageous

Negative aspects/ imbalance of this frequency:
Domineering, aggressive, obstinate, hatred, revenge, quick temper, resentful, fearful, and ruthless

Orange

Orange is next in the visible spectrum and has a frequency of 597nm. This color is associated with the body's muscular system, emotional health, and lower abdomen such as the uterus, large bowel, prostate, ovaries and testes. The endocrine glands are the ovaries and testes. Orange is connected to assisting the body to heal conditions of the stomach, pancreas, adrenal glands, and intestines. Too much orange can affect the nervous system. This can be balanced by introducing shades of green-blue. This color is good at removing negativity from the body; assisting with food digestion and elimination; influencing emotions, pleasure and desire; and stimulating creativity. Sunsets over the sea can appear to be more orange; that means there is more salt in the air. That means an excess of salt in the body can influence parts of the body functioning at the same frequency as red.

Positive aspects of this frequency:
Sociable, creativity, joyous, self confidence, constructive, independent, and enthusiastic

Negative aspects/ imbalance of this frequency:
Pride, dependency, destructive attitude, unsociable, and difficulty interacting with others

Yellow

Yellow has a frequency of 580nm and has higher photon energy, shorter wavelengths, and higher frequency than orange and red. The parts of the body associated with yellow include the liver, spleen, stomach and small intestines. The endocrine gland is the pancreas. Therefore yellow toxins are particularly harmful to these areas. This color relates to self-worth such as how we feel about ourselves. Yellow can be used for treating depression and digestive problems such as it helps to rebalance the entire gastrointestinal tract and elimination system. Too much yellow may lead to worry (excessive thinking), and nervousness. A sunset will appear yellow when the air is clear.

Positive aspects of this frequency:
Self-worth, good humored, logical, wisdom, confidence, and broad minded

Negative aspects/ imbalance of this frequency:
Cowardly, pessimistic, over analytical, vindictive, feelings of inferiority, and devious

Green

Green is in the middle of the spectrum and has a frequency of 527nm. It is the most dominant color on the planet and has the ability to balance and heal the body's energies. It is associated with the heart, circulatory, pulmonary and the autonomic nervous systems. The endocrine gland is the thymus (immune system). Green can sooth inflammation in the body and has a calming effect on the nervous system. This color has been associated with tissue regeneration and DNA repair, as well as being a strong influence on the development of an immature immune system. Green is the color of harmony and balance which can be used during times of stress. Green silk holds therapeutic effects to combat the aftermath of trauma.

Positive aspects of this frequency:
Generous, compassionate, harmonious, adaptable, practical, unconditional love, sympathetic, understanding, and to have a love of children, nature and animals

Negative aspects/ imbalance of this frequency:
Over-confident, miserly, jealous, angry, allowing others to take advantage of you, blaming others, hangs on to possessions, lack of consideration, indifferent, and unscrupulous with money

Blue

Blue has a frequency of 473nm, the wavelengths are shorter, the photon energy is higher, and the frequency is higher than the color green. The endocrine gland is the thyroid located in the throat. The upper digestive tract can be affected by an imbalance in this area. This frequency strongly affects the whole throat area including the esophagus, teeth, throat, thyroid and parathyroid glands, the respiratory system, and the entire vocal apparatus. As blue photons enter the earth's atmosphere, some of the shorter waves are eliminated by air, and blue light scatters in all directions giving the sky its blue color. Blue light covers a shorter distance; its waves are shorter, its energy is higher. Blue light is magnetic.

Positive aspects of this frequency:
Loyalty, trustworthy, peace, and tactful

Negative aspects/ imbalance of this frequency:
Cold, speaks negatively of others, resists change, clings to tradition, stubborn, slows to respond, surrenders to others, fanatical, and hyperactive

Sound

The Six Solfeggio Frequencies

1. UT   396 Hz: Liberates Guilt and Fear.
2. RE   417 Hz: Undoes Situations and Facilitates Change
3. MI   528 Hz: Transformation and Miracles,
               DNA repair and maintenance.
4. FA   639 Hz: Connection/Relationships.
5. SOL   741 Hz: Awakens Intuition
               Reconnection of the 12 strands of DNA, and
               self- truth. (Pineal Gland/Pituitary)
6. LA   852 Hz: Return to Spiritual Order.

Body/Organ	Hz	Musical Note
Thyroid/Parathyroid	492.8	B
Adrenal Glands	492.8	B
Pineal/Nerve pathways	448	A
Bones	418.3	Ab
Bladder	352	F
Blood	321.9	E
Muscles	324	E
Kidney	319.88	Eb
Liver	317.83	Eb
Intestines	281	C#
Mouth/Speech	263	D
Coccyx/Reproduction	256	C
Lungs	220	A
Colon	176	F
Stomach	110	A

Frequencies/Wavelengths in Association with the Body

295.8: Associated with fat cells (note: C#)
384: Mineral chromium (note: G)
396: Liberating Guilt and Fear Solfeggio Frequency 'UT' (note: G)
400: Mineral manganese (note: G)
405: Violet
417: Undo Situations and Facilitate Change Solfeggio Frequency 'RE'
418.3 Associated with bones (note: Ab)
438: Indigo
440: A (musical note)
448: Pineal Gland/Nerve Pathways (note: A)
464: Mineral copper (note: Bb)
473: Blue
480: Minerals phosphorous and zinc (note: B)
492: Associated with the spleen/intelligence
492.8: Associated with the adrenal glands
495: B (musical note)
526: Associated with top of the head and mouth
527: Green
528: C (musical note) 'MI' Transformation and Miracles Solfeggio Frequency
580: Yellow
586: Associated with sex and circulation (note: C#)
594: D (musical note)
600: Orange
639 Connection/Relationships 'FA' Solfeggio Frequency
658: Associated with nasal passages (breathing and taste)
660: E (musical note)
685: Associated with the ears
700: Red
704: F (musical note)
741: Awakening Intuition 'SOL' Solfeggio Frequency
787: Associated with the eyes
852: Return to Spiritual Order 'LA' Solfeggio Frequency
1000: Associated with cerebral neurons

Find out more: www.reactionhq.com.au

The Relationship between the Kidneys and the Lungs

Metabolic Water	Carbon Dioxide Gas
The kidneys regulate water and filter blood	Carbon dioxide gas is eliminated through the lungs

The filtration of water through the kidneys is dependent upon high oxygen arterial blood, that is, blood moving away from the heart. If the blood contains abnormal impurities such as a diet rich in unnatural, denatured, refined or processed foods, this extra oxygen is supplied by the adrenal glands. The adrenal glands' convenient location uses an internal supply of adrenoxidase to supply the kidneys with oxygen faster, so as to overcome any strain in the process taking place.

In the event of the adrenal glands being overtaxed, exhausted or weakened such that adrenal reserves are depleted, unable to facilitate the elimination of toxins through the kidney, the lungs try to help. They do this by secreting some of the toxins through their mucous. This in turn may cause inflammation or irritation in the lung region which, if the problem persists, may lead to respiratory problems such as asthma.

Cayenne pepper stimulates the *sympathetic* branch of the nervous system, which raises metabolism and thus helps the lungs by stimulating the removal of congestion and toxins from the system. Turmeric (yellow), the spice, also has medicinal properties used to cleanse the lungs. An apple a day is said to keep lungs healthy and increase their capacity.

Calcium

The kidneys and the parathyroid glands (located in the neck), regulate calcium metabolism.

The Calcium Paradox

o When less calcium is eaten in the diet, blood calcium levels may rise, including calcium found in many organs and tissues.
o Inflammation can lead to excessive uptake of calcium by cells. This is a factor in depression, obesity, and the degenerative diseases.
o When bones lose calcium the soft tissues calcify.

○   If an organ is deprived of calcium for a short length of time, it can lose its ability to take up normal amounts of calcium; thus, it can take up toxic levels instead.

Calcium and Cells

Magnesium and potassium are mainly intracellular (inside cells) whereas sodium and calcium are mainly extracellular (outside cells). When cells are stressed (they lack energy or get excited) magnesium and potassium are exchanged with sodium and calcium.

During stress, the mitochondria, the internal power plant of the cell, can bind to a certain amount of calcium. When this calcium builds to a certain point, it can inactivate the mitochondria, thus forcing the cell to increase its energy production, producing an excess of lactic acid. Dying or stressed cells take up calcium, exciting the cell at the same time, which intensifies stress. A cramp is an example of uncontrolled cellular excitation.

Prolonged excitation and stress can lead to tissue inflammation. Studies have shown that Vitamin D not only increases calcium absorption but it also plays an important role in anti-inflammation. Protein deficiency is an important factor behind abnormal calcium metabolism.

Science shows that the pineal gland has the highest calcium concentration of any normal soft tissue in the body and it calcifies with age. Calcification is the process in which calcium salts build up in soft tissue, causing it to harden. Pineal calcification over time can affect the brain's ability to function and can affect daily life tasks. Calcification is closely related to having a defective sense of direction and has been implicated in the onset of Multiple Sclerosis (MS).

A 1991 study by Sandyk R., and Awerbuch G.I,. published in the *International Journal of Neuroscience,* showed that pineal calcification was found in 100% of MS patients. Multiple Sclerosis tends to affect Caucasians disproportionately; it is nearly unheard of in Africa. Incidentally, the prevalence of peanut allergy in Africa is very low.

Calcium deficiency has been linked to hypertension (high blood pressure). Estrogen and oxygen deprivation can increase soft tissue calcium. Like magnesium, a calcium deficiency stimulates the parathyroid glands to produce more parathyroid hormone (PTH), to increase calcium absorption, which also removes calcium from the bones.

A calcium deficiency in the bones can affect bones, including the three small bones called "hammer" (malleus), "stirrup" (stapes), and "anvil" (incus), located in the middle ear. These delicate bones are involved in the mechanism of hearing and the sense of balance. Tinnitus, ringing or buzzing sounds in the ear, is the result of impaction of ear wax or inflammation of the eardrum or the middle ear. If symptoms such as lower back and joint pain and urinary problems exist, calcium absorption from a kidney imbalance may be the underlying cause of hearing problems.

Aspirin inhibits PTH action which helps to prevent calcification of inflamed tissues, and stop calcium loss from bones. Magnesium, progesterone, and many other substances are known to protect against excitotoxic calcium overload. Increased intracellular calcium, in conjunction with excess excitatory amino acids and nitric oxide, is involved in several neurodegenerative diseases.

Recommended Dietary Intake
Adults   800mg
Women over 54   1000mg
Pregnancy   1100mg
Breastfeeding   1200mg

Copper

Copper is a mineral required by the body for the production of bone and connective tissue, as well as to code specific enzymes that range in function from the removal of free radicals to the production of melanin. The stomach needs to be acidic in order to absorb copper. Therefore, high alkaline foods can interfere with the absorption of copper, as do milk and egg proteins. An environment high in copper can lead to vitamin E loss.

A copper deficiency can lead to joint pain, lower immune defense, osteoporosis, and because copper is essential for iron absorption, anemia. Too much copper can lead to short term cramps, vomiting and diarrhea. Long term copper toxicity can lead to depression, hypertension, schizophrenia, problems with memory, and insomnia. Too much zinc disrupts copper and iron absorption.

Recommended dietary intake
Adults   2mg

Ethanol

Ethanol, also called *pure*, *ethyl* or *drinking alcohol*, is a volatile, flammable, colorless liquid. It is the primary constituent used in alcoholic beverages; it is a central nervous system depressant; and it is metabolized by the body as an energy-providing nutrient. The human liver converts ethanol into acetaldehyde, which is more toxic than ethanol. This is then converted into harmless acetic acid by acetaldehyde dehydrogenase.

Acetaldehyde occurs widely in nature and is produced on a large scale industrially. It can be found in coffee, ripe fruit, bread, and is produced naturally by plants as part of their metabolism. For some, facial flushing may occur immediately after consuming alcohol; this is mainly seen in those of Asian descent. This temporary facial redness is known to be caused by an emzyme imbalance such as decreased activity of the *alcohol dehydrogenase* enzyme and possibly a missing enzyme called *aldehyde dehydrogenase*. What is important to note is the connection between facial redness and liver function.

Magnesium

Magnesium is directly involved in the healthy function of nerve cells, bone health, keeping the immune system healthy, maintaining a healthy heart rhythm, and it plays a role in hormone secretion. It is also involved in at least three hundred biochemical reactions throughout the body. Because magnesium is abundant in food, a deficiency is extremely rare. However, if a deficiency does occur, this can injure the heart and lead to cardiovascular disease or high blood pressure. A deficiency can also cause muscle spasms, diabetes, anxiety disorders, migraines, and osteoporosis.

A deficiency of magnesium stimulates the parathyroid glands to produce more parathyroid hormone, PTH, to increase calcium absorption, also removing calcium from the bones. Too much magnesium can lead to diarrhea as an attempt by the healing system to remove the excess. Magnesium is antagonistic to calcium because it is a basic protective calcium blocker.

Recommended dietary intake

Men	320mg
Women	270mg
Pregnancy	300mg
Breastfeeding	340mg

Potassium

Potassium (like sodium) plays a role in the regulation of fluid inside and outside the cells. It also plays a role in the healthy function of muscles and nerves. Too much potassium (found inside of cells) can lead to abnormal heart rhythms. Potassium is abundant in most food, thus, deficiency is rare but can occur due to diarrhea, vomiting, or kidney malfunction. Symptoms of potassium deficiency include fatigue and feeling unwell.

Recommended dietary intake
Adults   1950-5460mg

Sodium

Sodium is linked with potassium and regulates the flow of fluid in and out of cells. It is involved in muscle contractions and the transmission of nerve impulses. It is abundant in food and generally eaten in excess. Sodium (found in fluid outside of cells) when in excess for some can lead to hypertension, water retention, stress or damage the kidneys, and lead to congestive heart failure. Sodium chloride is better known as salt.

Chloride ions are secreted in gastric juice as hydrochloric acid, essential for food digestion. This is then absorbed by the intestines during digestion. Too much or too little sodium can cause cells to malfunction. Symptoms of a sodium deficiency may include dry mouth and tongue, low blood pressure, and problems with circulation. Because the kidneys receive twenty percent of the blood pumped by the heart, a sodium imbalance can injure the heart.

Recommended dietary intake
Adults   up to 2300mg

Sodium Benzoate (211)

This is an additive used as a food coloring and preservative in foods. High levels can create hyperactivity.

Zinc

Zinc is required by the body to maintain a strong immune system, and healthy eyes and skin. It also helps the body to heal (*parasympathetic* branch); it maintains a sense of smell, builds proteins, triggers enzymes, and creates DNA. It promotes growth and sexual development. Zinc also functions as a neurotransmitter helping cells to communicate.

Zinc deficiency can lower immune defense, cause hair loss, decrease appetite and taste, lower healing capabilities and cause night blindness.

Too much zinc can disrupt the absorption of copper and iron. It can also produce excessive amounts of toxic free radicals. Elevated copper in combination with low zinc levels has been associated with an explosive temper.

Recommended Dietary Intake
Adults   12mg
Pregnancy   16mg
Breastfeeding   18mg

Reaction!
Health Intelligence (HQ)

Hidden Factors

Aspartame: The Sweet Silent Killer

Phenylalanine in its synthetic form is better known as the artificial sweetener *aspartame* (food additive 951). Aspartame was discovered by accident in 1965 by James Schlatter, a chemist testing an anti-ulcer drug. Initially it was approved for use in dry foods in the middle of 1974; however, objections caused *aspartame* to be placed on hold six months later, awaiting FDA approval. By the early '80s *aspartame* was approved to use in dry goods and for use in carbonated beverages such as diet soda. Then a few years later, it was allowed in baked goods and confectionery.

In 1987, Professor Louis J. Elsas, II, M.D., made a statement before the U.S. Senate Committee during an investigation to determine if *aspartame* usage was safe for humans or not. He stated that studies prior had only ever been performed on rats whose metabolism of phenylalanine is more efficient than humans, and therefore rat studies were irrelevant. Despite this, by the mid '90s all restrictions from *aspartame* were lifted, allowing its usage in all foods.

Aspartame is a sweetener made from phenylalanine and the excitotoxin aspartate. Approval of aspartame surprised me when I dug deeper to find that this form of synthetic phenylalanine breaks down into several toxic and dangerous ingredients. Basically aspartame is poison, yet it is used to sweeten thousands of products today.

Label Watch:

Phenylalanine

Food additive 951

"Natural flavoring" can be a disguise for aspartame.

Sources of Aspartame

Diet soft drinks, sugar free chewing gum, children's medication, and other products that claim to be "diet", "low calorie", or "sugar free".

Aspartame is made up of three chemicals—aspartic acid (40%), phenylalanine (50%), and methanol (10%).

Aspartic Acid (40%)

Aspartic acid and glutamic acid (monosodium glutamate or MSG) act like neurotransmitters which in excess can kill certain neurons, allowing too much calcium into the cells. These chemicals are called "excitotoxins" because they can literally "excite" neurons to death. Excess amounts can seep through the blood brain barrier, which normally protects the brain from toxins in the blood.

As the brain is still in its infancy in childhood, these chemicals can be more damaging in the young. Incidentially, diet soda and other foods containing *aspartame* are heavily marketed to children.

Phenylalanine (50%)

Excess phenylalanine can decrease serotonin. Studies have shown that a build up in parts of the brain can lead to schizophrenia or seizures.

Methanol (10%)

Methanol is a deadly poison, gradually released when the ingested *aspartame* meets the enzyme chymotrypsin in the small intestine. This then breaks down into formic acid (ant venom) and formaldehyde (embalming fluid), a neurotoxin.

Formaldehyde is a carcinogen that can disrupt cell regeneration and cause birth defects. Methanol is extremely dangerous; it is known to cause blindness. Ethanol normally accompanies methanol as the antidote for methanol toxicity.

How Aspartame Harms the Body

According to medical researchers studying the adverse effects of *aspartame*, it can trigger a whole array of health and psychological disorders. Some of these symptoms include irrational mood swings, blurred vision, vertigo, tinnitus, problems with speech, loss of taste, asthma and chest tightness, nausea, weight gain, palpitations, panic attacks, brain lesions and tumors, memory loss, headaches, sleep disorders, muscle spasms or joint pains, sexually related problems, birth defects, depression, and skin problems.

It can also trigger diseases such as multiple sclerosis, Parkinson's disease, Alzheimer's disease, diabetes, chronic fatigue syndrome, and cancer in the lymphatic cells of the immune system.

Evidence has also shown that a byproduct of *aspartame* metabolism can lead to brain tumors, change cholesterol levels, and produce uterine polyps. Aspartame is known to be highly addictive.

As phenylalanine is a precursor for tyrosine, an amino acid used by the cells to synthesize proteins, dopamine, norepinephrine, epinephrine, and the skin pigment melanin, could an addiction to aspartame simply mean that this particular synthetic form of phenylalanine has been synthesized by the body into dopamine, a neurotransmitter that helps to control the brain's reward and pleasure center? If it had been synthesized into norepinephrine or epinephrine then symptoms may arise in the adrenal glands and surrounding areas. And if synthesized into melanin, then symptoms would appear in skin.

The acceptable dietary intake of aspartame
United States of America   50 mg
Australia/Europe   40 mg

Fluoride

Trace amounts of this dangerous chemical are found in the manufacture of dental products such as toothpaste, in drinking water, pesticides, and aluminium production. To some people it is a little disconcerting that the same fluoride used in drinking water is also a poison found in pesticides.

How Fluoride Harms the Body

A *soapy* taste can be associated with ingesting too much fluoride, otherwise known as sodium fluoride. This chemical can also be *absorbed through the skin such as through taking a bath or shower*. Chemicals absorbed through the skin are more dangerous because they enter the bloodstream more easily, and bypass the gut where they would normally bind with minerals from food which reduces any harmful effects. Fluoride ingestion interferes with many basic vital functions in the body by inhibiting enzyme activity, it interferes with oxygen usage by the cells, and it speeds up the body's breakdown of major structural protein collagen.

Fluoride can affect the pineal gland as well as cause hyperactivity, genetic mutations, damage red blood cells, cause muscle weakness and arthritis, a rare form of bone cancer in young males, Alzheimer's disease and other forms of dementia, birth defects, skeletal deformation, hypothyroidism, suppress thyroid function, lower IQ, impair immune function, cause infertility, early onset of puberty due to interference with the pineal gland, damage muscles, gastrointestinal problems, and cause kidney damage.

A study in India on fluoride-treated animals revealed that the animals produced less cortisol due to adrenocortical hypofunction. The study also revealed pituitary gland hypofunction, which is possibly the reason for adrenal insufficiency in the production of steroid hormones. India launched a Technology Mission on "Safe Drinking Water" in 1986 (now re-designated after the late Prime Minister Sh. Rajiv Gandhi as the Rajiv Gandhi National Drinking Water Mission) in which every drinking water source in the rural sector is checked for water quality, especially for fluoride.

As well as having high calcium levels, research in 1997 by Dr. Jennifer Luke from the University of Surrey in England showed that the pineal gland is the primary target of fluoride accumulation within the body, more so than teeth and bones. Fluoride reacts with calcium ions in the pineal gland to produce an insoluble substance.

"Fluorides are general protoplasmic poisons ...The sources of fluorine intoxication are drinking water containing 1 ppm or more of fluorine, fluorine compounds used as insecticidal sprays for fruits and vegetables and the mining and conversion of phosphate rock to superphosphate, which is used as fertilizer. The fluorine content of phosphate rock, about 25% of the fluorine present, is volatilized and represents a pouring into the atmosphere of approximately 25,000 tons of pure fluorine annually...The known effects of chronic fluorine intoxication are those of hypophasia of the teeth, which has been called mottled enamel, and of bone sclerosis." — *Journal of the American Medical Association*, September 18, 1943

According to toxicological profiles, those more susceptible to fluoride toxicity include the elderly, people with calcium, magnesium or vitamin C deficiencies, infants and young children, developing fetuses, diabetics, low thyroid function, people with kidney or heart problems, and pregnant women. Children are exposed to fluoride at an earlier age than fifty years ago. If the pineal accumulates fluoride at an earlier age than in previous decades, one would anticipate that a high local concentration of fluoride within the pineal would affect the functions of the pineal, i.e., the synthesis of hormonal products, specifically melatonin. *Silver Colloid* not only sanitizes water, research has shown that it reacts with fluoride before it hits the calcium in the pineal gland.

Melamine

Melamine is a nitrogen-based compound used in industrial plastics, such as eating utensils and laminates (kitchenware), flooring, whiteboards and flame retardant fabrics. According to the U.S. Food and Drug Administration (FDA), it is also used as a fertilizer in Asia and a metabolite of the pesticide cyromazine. Some Chinese food companies have been found to use melamine in wheat flour and other food products such as baby formula because it makes the food appear to have more protein. Therefore, some cheap protein supplements on the market may contain this nitrogen-based compound. Melamine can result in kidney stones and kidney disorder due to melamine crystals and other by-products forming in the urine and kidneys.

Vaccinations/Immunization

Vaccines are not just made up of the viruses and diseases that should or should not be present, but they are filled with a host of cellular debris from non-humans: from monkeys, chickens, and even cancer cells. These can contain foreign DNA and RNA genetic codes, enzymes, proteins, and chemicals.

According to the U.S. Protection Agency, safe exposure to mercury is 0.1 microgram per kilogram of body weight per day, yet fully vaccinated children receive up to 237.5 micrograms of mercury from vaccines in a dose of 25 micrograms each. Mercury exposure has been linked to neurological disorders, including possibly autism. Some vaccine cultures also contain trypsin. Rarely is the patient's immune system checked for suppression or deficiency prior to inoculation.

Raw Food versus Cooked Food

Enzymes play a major role in digestion and other bodily functions. Raw food contains half the amount of enzymes required to break itself down during digestion however these are destroyed when the food or drinks are heated above 115°F. This can place extra stress on the body to use up its own metabolic enzymes. About half of essential amino acids (building block for protein) coagulate at temperatures reaching over 115°F which makes them unusable, thus carcinogenic.

Fat turns into hydrogenated fat also above 115°F which makes these fat unusable carcinogens. Heat destroys water-soluble vitamins making them toxic and thus adds stress to the immune system. Carbohydrates carbonize and caramelize when cooked at high temperatures.

Food, water and air all contain oxygen. Cancer and many other diseases cannot exist in an adequately oxygenated environment. Cooked food and animal products put more of a demand on the body for oxygen to metabolize. Live raw food contains its own paramagnetic field which the body's electrical field benefits from. Basically live food adds a paramagnetic charge to the body which increases its life force.

Nobel Prize winner Dr. Popp discovered that the human body retains, absorbs and emits light energy (photons), that 97% of human DNA gives off photons. Photons are absorbed from food and drinks to fuel its bio-electric field. When food is cooked, the dead matter must be filled with photons for the body to assimilate the food. This in turn weakens the body. Research has shown that cancer thrives on cooked food where the light has dimmed, and dies off in a live food environment when light is radiant.

Source	When cooked
Oils and Fats found in food	Toxins: Ally aldehyde, Nitrobenzene, Nitropyrene and Butyric acid
Sugars	Toxins: Furans, Furfurals
Fat from milk, eggs, fish and meat	Toxins: Unsaturated Aldehydes Epoxides
Peanuts (roasted)	Allergens: Ara h1 and Ara h2

Peanut

Peanuts have a variety of industrial uses. They are used in the production of lubricating oil, paint, leather dressing, varnish, furniture polish, and insecticides. Nitroglycerin is made from peanut oil; some soaps and many cosmetics contain peanut oil derivatives. Its protein is used in the manufacturing of some textiles. Peanut shells have been used in the manufacture of abrasives and glue, fuel, wallboard, and plastic. It is also one of the main ingredients used in dynamite.

According to a study done in 2003, roasting peanuts, a common occurrence in North America, causes the peanut allergen Ara h2 to become a stronger trypsin inhibitor, thus making the peanut more resistant to digestion. Another peanut allergen Ara h1 also becomes more resistent to digestion through the process of roasting.

One could theorize that the immune system could perceive a strong trypsin inhibitor as a threat, especially if there is an imbalance of trypsin or derivatives thereof, either too much or too little in the body's internal environment.

Trypsin Inhibitors

Trypsin inhibitors are chemicals that reduce the availability of trypsin in the body. There are four commercial sources of trypsin inhibitors:

1. Serum Antitrypsin, also called serum trypsin inhibitor.
2. Lima beans; there are six lima bean inhibitors.
3. Ovomucoid; found in raw avian egg white.
4. Soybeans; found in soybean. Chymotrypsin is also inhibited by this chemical.
5. Bovine pancreas; this chemical is a pancreatic inhibitor. Chymotrypsin is also inhibited by this chemical.

Label Watch:
Contain Peanut:

Arachis hypogaea
Arachis oil
Artificial nuts
Cold pressed, extruded, or
expelled peanut oil
Beer nuts
Crushed nuts, crushed peanuts
Earth nuts
Dry roasted peanuts
Goober peas
Goobers
Ground nuts
Ground peanuts
Hydrolyzed peanut protein
Hypogaeic acid

Mandelonas
Mixed nuts
Monkey nuts
Nut pieces
Nutmeat
Peanuts
Peanut butter
Peanut butter chips
Peanut butter morsels
Peanut flour
Peanut paste
Peanuts sauce
Peanut syrup
Satay
Spanish peanuts
Virginia peanuts

May Contain Peanut:

Artificial flavoring
Baked goods
Cakes, Candy and Chocolate
Cereals
Chili
Cocktails / Some alcoholic drinks
Cosmetics
Crumb toppings
Desserts
Ethnic foods: African, Asian,
Chinese, Indian, Indonesian, Thai,
Vietnamese, Mexican
Food additive 322
Fried foods
Flavoring

Gravy
Hydrolyzed plant protein
Hydrolyzed vegetable protein
Lupine is a legume that cross-
reacts with peanut
Marzipan
Mole sauce
Natural flavoring
Nut paste
Nougat
Pesto
Pet food
Personal hygiene products (soap)
Salad dressings
Waldorf Salad

Latin Translation of Allergens

Allergen	Latin
Almond (Bitter)	Prunus Amara
Almond (Sweet)	Prunus Dulcis
Brazil	Bertholetia Excelsa
Cod Liver Oil	Gadi Iecur
Egg	Ovum
Hazelnut	Corylus Rostrata, Americana, or Avellana
Milk	Lac
Mixed Fish Oil	Piscum Iecur
Peanut	Arachis Hypogaea
Sesame	Sesamum Indicum
Walnut	Juglans Regia or Juglans Nigra

Furfurals

Furfurals are an organic compounds derived from agricultural byproducts of wheat bran, oats, corncob, sugarcane, and sawdust. It has a colorless oily liquid, which turns *yellow* when exposed to air, and also has an almond-like odor. When furfurals are heated in the presence of acid it irreversibly solidifies into a resin. Although furfurals appear in many foods and flavorants, it is toxic. Furfurals are known to irritate the skin. Chronic exposure can lead to a skin allergy and increase susceptibility to sunburn.

Nitrobenzene

Nitrobenzene is a water-soluble *yellowish* oil that is highly toxic when used in large quantities. It has an almond-like odor and can also be absorbed through the skin. It is sometimes used as a flavoring or as an additive in perfume. It is also used in shoe and floor polish, paint solvent, and to mask unpleasant odors such as in an inexpensive perfume for soap.

Prolonged exposure of nitrobenzene may lead to the following; vision impairment, liver, kidney or central nervous system damage, anemia, and lung irritation. Ingestion or inhalation may induce headaches, fatigue, arms and legs weakness, dizziness, nausea, vomiting, irritate the gastrointestinal tract, or even cause internal bleeding. The United Stated Environmental Protection Agency has classified nitrobenzene as a likely human carcinogen.

Unsaturated Aldehydes

The simplest form of unsaturated aldehyde is acrolein, known for its unpleasant, acrid odor such as the smell of burnt fat (when cooking oil reaches smoke point). Acrolein is formed when glycerol in burning fat breaks down. It can also be produced by the reaction of potassium bisulfate on glycerol when heated. Acrolein is used in the preparation of acrylic acid, polyester (resin) and polyurethane. It is also used as a contact herbicide to control weeds and algae in irrigation canals.

If acrolein is left at room temperature it has a tendency to polymerize into a gummy *yellowish* residue which has a strong unpleasant odor. Acrolein severely irritates the respiratory system; an agent used in tear gas. It was used as a chemical weapon (in a more toxic form) in World War I. A connection has been linked to cigarette smoke and lung cancer; bladder infections/inflammation; and may assist in the development of multiple sclerosis because it can damage myelin nerve sheaths.

Glycerol (or glycerin, glycerine) is central to all lipids (fats are a subgroup of lipids called triglycerides). The main function of lipids include energy storage, they form structural components of cells, and act as important signaling molecules.

More Hidden Factors

By increasing your health intelligence (HQ), you are in a better position to make some changes in your life to quench some of the fires within. This in turn gives the internal healer more control to restore balance.

Reaction! Health Intelligence HQ

Please visit my website to find out more about products, process work, and/or resources mentioned in this book. Also, to learn more about my accredited anaphylaxis and first aid courses and health intelligence workshops which have been specifically formulated to incorporate my own first-hand experience and health intelligence acquired over a lifetime from living with a potentially life-threatening condition to living without it.

www.reactionhq.com.au

Make Sense of your own Invisible Enemy

REACTI◎N HQ
Health Intelligence for Life
www.reactionhq.com.au

Bibliography

As my quest to find answers has spanned over a lifetime of research, I have made every effort to complete this bibliography as accurately as possible.

American Peanut Council. *About the Peanut Industry*
(http://www.peanutsusa.com)
Australasian Society for Clinical Immunology and Allergy (ASCIA).
Economic Impact of Allergies -- Report (Access Economics, 2007)
Baconnier, Lang et al. *Bioelectromagnetics "Calcite Microcrystals in the Pineal Gland of the Human Brain -- First Physical and Chemical Studies."* (2002)
Batmanghelidj, F., M.D. *Your Body's Many Cries for Water: You Are Not Sick, You Are Thirsty!* (Global Health Solutions, Inc., 1995)
Baumeister, R. F. and Tice, D. M. *Anxiety and Social Exclusion*
(Journal of Social and Clinical Psychology, 1990)
BBC Health News. *Peanut allergy diagnoses 'higher in boys'*
(http://www.bbc.co.uk, 2010)
Becker, Robert, M.D., and Marino, Andrew, Ph.D. *Electromagnetism & Life* (State University of New York, 1982)
Barker, Robin. *The Mighty Toddler*
(Pan Macmillan Australia Pty Ltd., Australia, 2001)
Bayliss C.R., Bishop N.L., and Fowler R.C. *Pineal gland calcification and defective sense of direction* Br Med J (Clin Res Ed, 1985)
Braden, Gregg. *The Isaiah Effect: Decoding the Lost Science of Prayer and Prophecy* (Harmony Books, U.S., 2000)
Bradshaw, John. *Healing The Shame That Binds You* (Health Communications, Inc., Florida, 1988)
—. *Home Coming: Reclaiming and Championing Your Inner Child*
(Bantam Books, U.S. and Canada, 1992)
Braiker, Harriet B, Ph.D. *The Disease to Please* (McGraw-Hill, U.S., 2001)
Brownstein, Art, M.D. *Extraordinary Healing – The Amazing Power of Your Body's Secret Healing System* (Harbor Press, Inc., 2005)
Chopra, Deepak, M.D. *Quantum Healing*
(Bantam Books, New York, 1989)
—. *Ageless Body, Timeless Mind* (Harmony Books, New York, 1993)
—. *Perfect Health* (Bantam Books, 1990)
Cloud, John. *Why Your DNA Isn't Your Destiny*
(Time Magazine Health, 2010)

Edelman, Susan, Ph.D. *Change Your Thinking*
(ABC Books, Australia, 2002)

Gamlin, Linda. *The Allergy Bible*
(Quadrille Publishing Limited, London, 2001)

Glasser, George. *Fluoride: A Toxic Tort Perspective* (1996)

Gregory, Richard L. *The Oxford Companion to The Mind*
(Oxford University Press, New York, 1987)

Grove, B. *Drinking Ourselves to Death?* (Newleaf, 2001)

Giacomo Rizzolatti et al. *Premotor cortex and the recognition of motor actions*
(Cognitive Brain Research, 1996)

Goleman, Daniel. *Social Intelligence* (Hutchinson, London, 2006)

Gyurak, A., and Ayduk, O. *Defensive physiological reactions to rejection: The
effect of self esteem and attentional control on startle responses.*
(Psychological Science, 2007)

Hadady, L. *Herbal Secrets for Total Health, The Complete Guide to Asian
Herbal Medicine* (Random House, London, UK, 1997)

Harrison, Eric *The Naked Buddha Second Edition*
(Perth Meditation Centre, Australia, 1999)

Harrison, Yvonne. *Sleep Talking* (Blandford, U.K., 1999)

Hawking, Stephen M. *A Brief History of Time* (Bantam, 1988)

Horowitz, L., and Puleo, J. *Healing Codes for the Biological Apocalypse.*
(Tetrahedron Publishing Group, 1999)

Kaptchuk, T.J. *Chinese Medicine, The Web that has no Weaver*
(Random House Ltd., London, U.K., 1997)

Kormondy, Edward J., and Essenfeld, Bernice E. *Biology*
(Addison-Wesley Publishing Company, U.S. and Canada, 1984)

King, Petrea. *Quest For Life*
(Random House Australia Pty Ltd., Australia, 2004)

Koukkari, W.L., and Sothern, R.B. *Introducing Biological Rhythms*
(Springer, New York, 2006)

Kross, Ethan, Berman, Marc G., Mischel, Walter, Smith, Edward E.,
and Wager, Tor D. *Social rejection shares somatosensory representations with
physical pain* (Proceedings of the National Academy of Sciences, 2011)

Larre, Claude, and de la Vallée, Elizabeth *Chinese Medicine from the Classics: the Seven Emotions – Psychology and Health in Ancient China* (China Books, 1996)

Laurie, Sanders G., and Tucker, Melvin J. *Centering: The Power of Meditation* (Excalibur Books, U.K., 1982)

Law Nolte, Dorothy, and Harris, Rachel. *Children Learn What They Live.* (Finch Publishing Pty, Ltd, Australia and New Zealand, 2008)

Lung and Asthma Information Agency (LAIA). *http://www.laia.ac.uk/asthma.htm*

Maestroni G.J. *The immunoneuroendocrine role of melatonin* (J Pineal Res., 1993)

Mayo Clinic, The. *Allergen Avoidance* (http://www.mayoclinic.com)

McEvoy, J.P., and Zarate, Oscar. *Introducing Quantum Theory* (Allen & Unwin Pty Ltd, Australia, 2004)

McKeown, Thomas. *The Origins of Human Disease* (Blackwell Pub, 1988)

Millman, Dan. *No Ordinary Moments* (H J Kramer Books and New World Library, U.S., 1992)

Mirror, The. *Pregnant mothers could be sensitising their unborn children by eating peanut-based foods (U.K., 1995)*

Murphy, Joseph, Dr. *The Power of Your Subconscious Mind* (Bantam, New York, 2001)

Noontil, Annette. *The Body Is The Barometer Of The Soul – So Be Your Own Doctor II* (Rainbow Spirit, 1996)

O'Connor, Dermot. *The Healing Code* (Hodder Headline Ireland and Hodder & Stoughton, 2006)

Pert, Candace B., Ph.D. *Molecules of Emotion: Why You Feel the Way You Do* (Scribner, New York, 2003)

Reader's Digest Sydney. *Strengthen Your Immune System* (Reader's Digest (Australia) Pty Limited, Australia and New Zealand, 2010)

Rees, Martin. *Just Six Numbers: The Deep Forces That Shape The Universe* (Basic Books, U.S., 2000)

Revill, Jo. *Allergy Explosion* (Kyle Cathie Limited, U.K., 2007)

Roberts, Janine. *Fear of the Invisible* (Impact Investigative Media Productions, 2008)

Schwarz, Jack. *Human Energy Systems* (E.P. Dutton, New York, 1980)

Stein, M., Mendelsohn, J., Obermeyer, W.H., Amromin, J., and Benca, R. *Sleep and Behavior Problems in School-Aged Children* (Pediatrics April 2001)

Sigelman, Carol K., and Rider, Elizabeth A. *Life-Span Human Development* (Thomson Wadsworth, Canada, 2006)

Sisgold, Steve. *What's Your Body Telling You?* (McGraw-Hill, U.S., 2009)

Sither Bradley, Tamdin, Dr. *Tibetan Medicine* (Thorsons, 2000)

Shostak, M. *Nisa: The life and words of a !Kung woman* (Random House, 1981)

Yiamouyiannis, John, Dr. *Fluoride the Aging Factor* (Health Action Press, 1986)

Wikipedia, the free encyclopedia

Williams, Kipling D., Joseph P. Forgas, and William von Hippel *The Social Outcast: Ostracism, Social Exclusion, Rejection, and Bullying* (Psychology Press, 2005)

Wolfe, David. *The Sunfood Diet Success System* (North Atlantic Books, 1999)

Young, Michael C, M.D. *The Peanut Allergy Answer Book* (Fair Winds, U.S., 2001)

Be a part of the
REACTI☉N Hꝴ
COMMUNITY

Sharing your story can really
Make a Huge Difference

Send your own health success story to
michelle@reactionhq.com.au

Join on Facebook:
www.facebook.com/Reaction20MinutestoLive

Follow on Twitter:
www.twitter.com/ReactionHQ

REACTI☉N Hꝴ
Health Intelligence for Life
www.reactionhq.com.au

What is Anaphylaxis?

Anaphylaxis is the most acute form of allergic reaction that can be fatal. It must be treated as an emergency that requires immediate treatment and urgent medical attention.

Symptoms of an acute allergic reaction or anaphylaxis:

The body may be engulfed in hives or an itchy rash. The face, lips, eyes, and tongue may swell; the airways narrow; the person may find it hard to breathe, they may experience nausea, vomiting, and diarrhea, and a sudden drop in blood pressure.

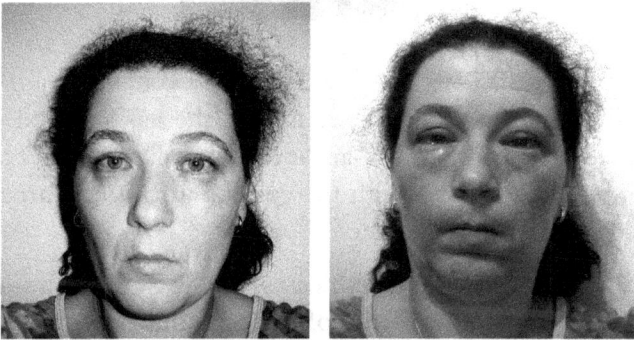

Courtesy of Michelle Flanagan: Photographs of an anaphylactic reaction.

Photographs from left to right: Author, Michelle Flanagan experiencing the early signs of an allergic reaction approximately five minutes after applying moisturizer to her face. The product did not have 'peanuts' listed on the label. The photograph on the right was taken approximately ten minutes later. Michelle was in an ambulance on her way to the nearest emergency room to receive urgent medical attention not long thereafter.

Common triggers of anaphylaxis:

Food such as peanuts, tree nuts, milk, eggs, fish, shellfish, sesame, soy and wheat; **Insect stings/bites** such as bee, wasp and jack jumper ant; **Medications** of both over the counter and prescribed; **latex**; and sometimes **exercise**.

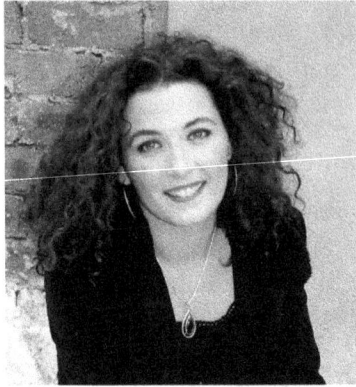

About the Author

Michelle Flanagan is truly unique in that she has suffered with, and healed herself of Anaphylaxis—an 'incurable' allergy that can lead to death. Not only did she live with the condition for over three decades, she has also lived without it since 2006.

In 2004, Michelle reached a health crisis. She was only thirty-five years old when faced with the threat of cancer and Grave's disease—an autoimmune disease of the thyroid gland. Limited by treatment choices due to multiple deadly allergies (peanut, shellfish, penicillin, and insect venom), she embarked on a remarkable journey deep inside the world of anaphylaxis seeking answers. This is where she would find the path to freedom and perfect health—without life threatening illness.

Michelle is a certified trainer, public speaker, and Master Practitioner of Neuro-Linguistic Programming (NLP), accredited by the International Hypnosis Association. She has a lifetime of experience on conquering almost impossible challenges; has formally studied food and nutrition; has traveled the world despite limitations that came with deadly consequences; has volunteered as Travel Officer for the anaphylaxis support group in Australia (1998 - 2001); and has been an Australian accredited Anaphylaxis and First Aid Trainer since 2009, facilitating nationally recognized courses and workshops that embody her own first-hand personal experience and rare perspective on living with and then without a life-threatening health condition.

Through the unique journey outlined in this book, Michelle shares a wealth of knowledge learned over a lifetime.

www.ingramcontent.com/pod-product-compliance
Lightning Source LLC
Chambersburg PA
CBHW070716280326
41926CB00087B/2247